(3

D0962467

WEED

THE USER'S GUIDE

WEED

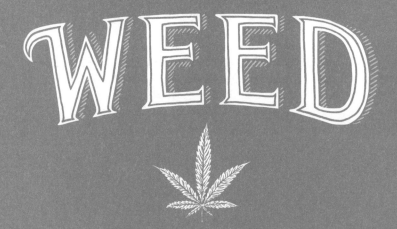

THE USER'S GUIDE

A 21ST CENTURY HANDBOOK FOR ENJOYING MARIJUANA

DAVID SCHMADER

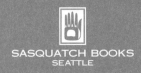

SASQUATCH BOOKS
SEATTLE

Printed in the United States of America

Published by Sasquatch Books
20 19 18 17 16   9 8 7 6 5 4 3 2 1

Editor: Hannah Elnan
Production editor: Emma Reh
Illustration: Alex DeSpain
Design: Joyce Hwang
Copyeditor: Nancy W. Cortelyou

Library of Congress Cataloging-in-Publication Data is available.

ISBN: 978-1-63217-042-2

Sasquatch Books
1904 Third Avenue, Suite 710
Seattle, WA 98101
(206) 467-4300
www.sasquatchbooks.com
custserv@sasquatchbooks.com

Certified Chain of Custody
Promoting Sustainable Forestry
www.sfiprogram.org
SFI-01268

SFI label applies to the text stock

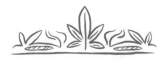

This book is dedicated to weed dealers, whose legal risk-taking allows so many of us to enjoy the miraculous effects of marijuana, which are pleasurable enough to make up for those dealers who insist on giving lectures on Chem Trails before handing over the goods. Most importantly, this book is dedicated to every American imprisoned for nonviolent marijuana possession, whose fate must be rectified through legislative action if legal marijuana is ever to be considered a truly guilt-free pleasure.

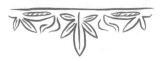

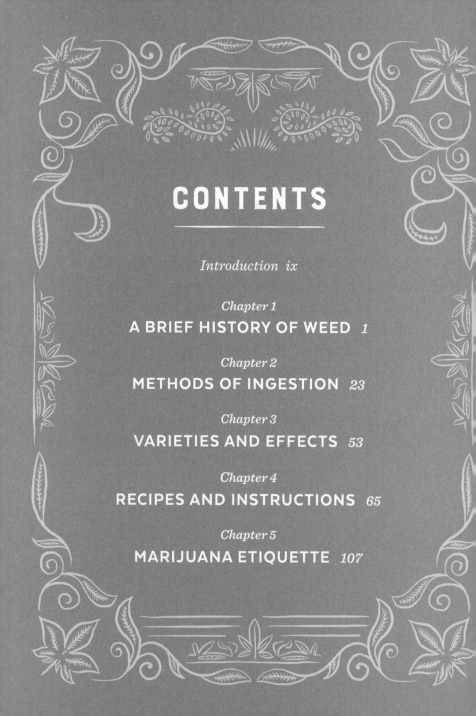

CONTENTS

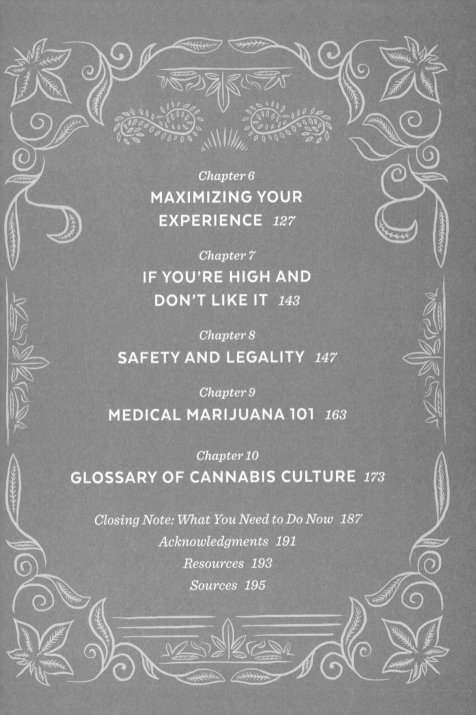

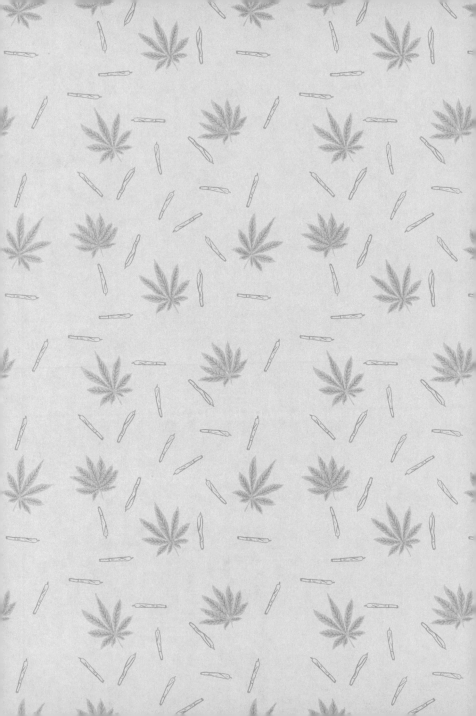

INTRODUCTION

The life-enhancing potential of marijuana first made itself known to me when I was nineteen. A group of friends and I were headed out to a Mexican restaurant, and en route one friend whipped out a joint and passed it around. I'd smoked weed before and enjoyed it. I'd eaten Mexican food before and enjoyed it. But the combination of the two was revelatory. One of weed's great powers is sensory enhancement, and my sensory-enhanced encounter with a nothing-fancy enchilada plate was a full-immersion Technicolor opera starring pico de gallo–soaked rice and delicious bits of charred cheese around the edges. When I was done, I felt like I'd just had a short face-to-face with God in my mouth.

This enchilada epiphany led me to further investigation of weed's power to enrich sensory perception and facilitate immersive engagement with the world. I was thrilled to find it worked with music (I spent what felt like hours swimming around in the space between notes on Cowboy Junkies' languorous *The Trinity Session*), comedy (ditto sob-laughing through compulsive replays of *30 Rock*'s "Werewolf Bar Mitzvah"), and conversation.

Still, the fact remained that all these seriously enriching pleasures were forbidden—banned by law and disparaged by society, the majority of which lazily adhered to the stereotype of potheads as basement-dwelling burnouts on the level of the fictional Cheech & Chong.

But what about all the high-functioning, life-loving adults—doctors, lawyers, engineers, entrepreneurs, authors, parents—who comprise the vast majority of weed smokers I know? The reality of responsible adult marijuana use is a fact of life that's ever more apparent, thanks in large part to citizen-driven efforts to reclassify, decriminalize, and legalize marijuana. This book is a guide for all those interested in exploring the wide, wonderful, post-"War on Drugs"-terror-hyperbole world of marijuana.

That all sounds great but perhaps you're wondering: Does weed require a "user's guide"? Aren't the basic facts known to every middle-school rebel puffing behind a Dumpster?

Yes and no. (But mostly no.)

Yes, marijuana's ability to produce psychoactive effects in human users is common knowledge. But beyond this fact lies a world of nuance and discernment that I will map in this book—synthesizing information from the existing pool of marijuana wisdom and offering myself up as an experienced test subject and tour guide. (Another reason for a user's guide is that today's concentrated marijuana products are a far cry from the grassy stuff folks might've smoked at Woodstock or in the '80s in college—a fact that makes even past personal experience an unfortunately unreliable guide to twenty-first-century weed.)

In this book, you'll find all you need to know to about the current state of recreational marijuana, from methods of ingestion and varieties of effects to edible recipes and tips for maximizing your marijuana experience.

What you won't find in this book is reckless encouragement to smoke marijuana. Even among people who love it, experiences of being high differ widely, and there are tons of folks who just don't enjoy the sensations marijuana offers. To these people, I offer my sympathies, my support, and Chapter 7: If You're High and Don't Like It.

To everyone else, a final bit of wisdom from Stephen Colbert, who delivered this gem at the end of a scared-straight drug lecture on *Strangers with Candy*: "All I'm saying is, if you still want to smoke pot, then be prepared to spend a lot of time laughing with your friends."

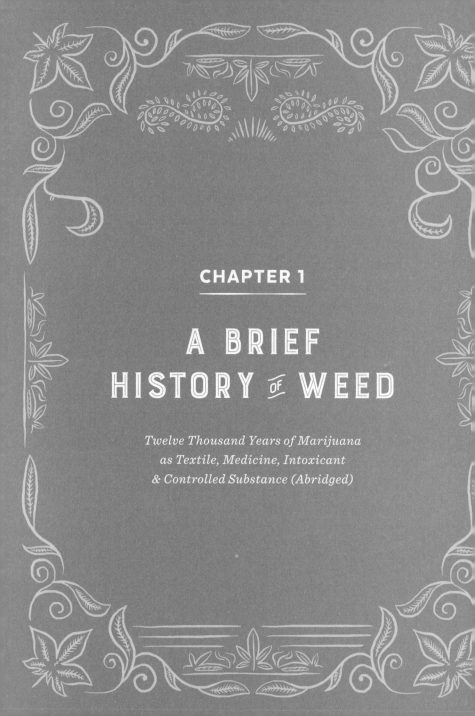

CHAPTER 1

A BRIEF HISTORY *of* WEED

*Twelve Thousand Years of Marijuana
as Textile, Medicine, Intoxicant
& Controlled Substance (Abridged)*

The history of weed begins roughly twelve thousand years ago, when the first cannabis plant pushed its spiky leaflets up through the grasslands of the Eurasian steppe. Pollinated by wind and coddled by humidity, the cannabis plant spread eastward, where it was initially appreciated for the strong fiber of its stalk, which became known as hemp. The first documented use of the plant comes from what is now Taiwan, where ancient pottery makers bolstered their clay with hemp-fiber cord.

Over the next nine thousand years, the use of cannabis as a textile spread westward, with the passage of time bringing increased refinement. In 1500 BCE, central Eurasian Scythians used hemp fiber to weave a linen-like cloth, and in 100 BCE, the Chinese created the first hemp paper.

Meanwhile, humans were steadily awakening to cannabis's supplementary uses, led by Chinese Emperor Fu Hsi, who in 2900 BCE declared weed to be medicine infused with both yin and yang, making it helpful for restoring balance, as well as minimizing the painful effects of gout, rheumatism, and menstruation. Over the next two centuries, medical cannabis spread to Egypt, India, and the Middle East, gaining praise as an aid for seemingly everything, from improving judgment to curing leprosy. (More prosaic ancient uses include as a sleep aid, appetite enhancer, and general anesthetic.) By 1 CE, a Chinese pharmacopoeia would recommend cannabis for over one hundred ailments.

DID CANNABIS CREATE CIVILIZATION?

This question was floated by celebrity astronomer Carl Sagan in his Pulitzer-winning book *The Dragons of Eden: Speculations on the Evolution of Human Intelligence.* Riffing on African Pygmies' long-standing habit of growing cannabis, Sagan wrote, "It would be wryly interesting if in human history the cultivation of marijuana led generally to the invention of agriculture, and thereby to civilization." Wryly interesting it may be, but factual it is not, as agriculture's founder crops remain emmer and einkorn wheat. Perhaps a better question is, did cannabis create Carl Sagan? Over the course of his career, Sagan sang marijuana's praises as loudly as a government-funded scientist dare, citing weed's enhancement of creativity and intellectual engagement, arguing in favor of medical marijuana, and writing politely confrontational letters to the Reagan Administration about its disingenuous vilification of weed. As Sagan wrote in a 1969 essay "Mr. X," "The illegality of cannabis is outrageous, an impediment to full utilization of a drug which helps produce the serenity and insight, sensitivity and fellowship so desperately needed in this increasingly mad and dangerous world."

As for mind-altering weed usage, the pioneer prize goes to the Scythians, the eastern Iranian equestrian tribes that populated the central Eurasian steppe starting in 8000 BCE. Their cannabis habits were documented by the Greek historian Herodotus in 440 BCE: "The Scythians, as I said, take some of this hemp-seed and, creeping under the felt coverings, throw it upon the red-hot stones; immediately it smokes, and gives out such a vapour as no Grecian vapour-bath can exceed; the Scyths, delighted, shout for joy." (Thank you, Scyths, for inventing the hot box, see glossary entry on page 180.)

Other early adopters of cannabis as a gateway to the sublime were the ancient Hindus of India and Nepal, whose sacred text the Atharvaveda praised "the wise drinking of bhang"—a concoction made of milk and cannabis—as a means to become one with Shiva. (However, Hindus believed "foolish" drinking of bhang—use outside of religious ritual—was a soul-diminishing sin.)

Cannabis continued to flourish as a textile as industrial hemp use spread across Europe. By 1533 CE, hemp ropes and sailcloth were in such demand in England that King Henry VIII commanded landowners to devote a certain percentage of their acreage to cannabis cultivation—or be fined.

In the early seventeenth century, the English settlers of Jamestown brought cannabis with them to the Americas, harvesting hemp to make rope and clothing. By 1762, the Colony of Virginia was awarding bounties for hemp production and penalizing those who shirked their hempy duty. By the start of the nineteenth century, cannabis plantations flourished in New York, Georgia, South Carolina, Mississippi, Nebraska, Kentucky, and California.

Medicinal use of cannabis also continued to expand. By 200 CE, Chinese physician Hua Tuo was anesthetizing surgery patients with a mix of cannabis resin and wine. In 1621's *The Anatomy of Melancholy*, English clergyman

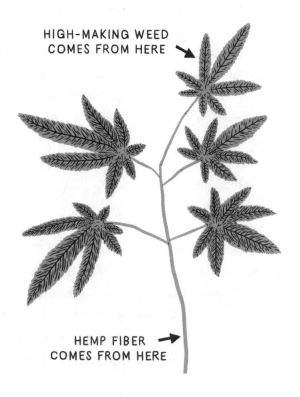

HIGH-MAKING WEED
COMES FROM HERE

HEMP FIBER
COMES FROM HERE

Robert Burton recommended cannabis as a treatment for depression. In 1753, Swedish botanist Carl Linnaeus first classified the cannabis plant with taxonomic nomenclature (*Cannabis sativa*), and in 1842, cannabis found its place in mainstream British medicine, thanks to Irish physician Dr. William O'Shaughnessy, who popularized its use for a variety of ailments, including menstrual cramps, muscle spasms, and convulsions brought on by epilepsy, tetanus, and rabies. The United States followed Britain's lead, and by 1850, patented cannabis products were easily purchased in general stores and used to treat everything from tonsillitis to alcoholism.

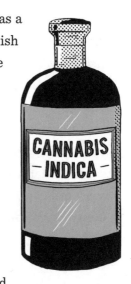

As medicinal use grew, so did spiritual/recreational use. In the tenth century, the habit of eating hashish for its psychotropic effects spread throughout Arabia, with Sufis using hash as a means of kick-starting mystical consciousness and enhancing the ability to appreciate the nature of Allah. Meanwhile, non-Sufis enjoyed hash for its powers of inebriation. One story in the Arabic collection *One Thousand and One Nights* calls cannabis "that hilarious herb" and "that jocund influence," while acknowledging that getting too high can inspire odd behavior like fishing in the middle of the night and urinating on your friends. (Seriously, look it up.)

In the seventeenth century, hashish grew into a major trade item across Asia, and in the eighteenth century, hash got its first major pushback, as French soldiers returning from Egypt brought that country's hash-eating habit home with them, inspiring Napoleon—who apparently resented Frenchmen adopting a habit favored by the Egyptian lower classes—to declare total prohibition against cannabis in France.

Cannabis continued to flourish across Africa in the nineteenth century, culminating with the Bashilenge tribe of the Congo. In 1881, the Bashilenge established the Riamba cult, whose members called themselves "the sons of hemp," of which they partook regularly, ascribing all sorts of magical and evil-combating powers to their beloved weed. By the end of the nineteenth century, the India Hemp Drugs Commission Report clocked the legal import of seventy thousand kilograms of hashish per year into India from central Asia.

Things took a sharp turn in the twentieth century. In 1906, the US Congress passed the Pure Food and Drug Act, which effectively classified cannabis and all other narcotics as poisons, attainable only at pharmacies with a doctor's prescription. Within a decade, California passed an amendment to make possession of "extracts, tinctures, or other narcotic preparations of hemp, or loco-weed" a misdemeanor, inspiring similar laws in Colorado, Louisiana,

WAS JESUS A STONER?

The answer to this question is as twisty and conditional as religion itself. It begins in the original Hebrew version of the Book of Exodus, which features a recipe for holy anointing oil that calls for over six pounds of kaneh-bosem, an aromatic grass that's been identified by several reputable botanists and linguists as cannabis. According to lore, early anointing rituals involved more than just an oily thumb swipe across the forehead—subjects were drenched in oil, the explicit purpose of which was to sanctify the anointed one as "most holy." As for Jesus Christ, "Christ" translates to "the anointed one," which suggests that Jesus came into contact with holy weed oil at least once. So, if Jesus indeed underwent a full-drench anointing with cannabis-infused oil, he may have once gotten very high. However, most reputable botanists and linguists identify kaneh-bosem not as cannabis but sweet cane and/or Indian lemongrass, in which case Jesus probably never got stoned, but for a while he smelled as beautiful as his ideals.

Maine, Massachusetts, Nevada, New York, Texas, Utah, Vermont, and Wyoming. Other nations followed suit, with the 1920s bringing regulation of non-medicinal cannabis to the United Kingdom, New Zealand, and Lebanon, with Canada following in 1923.

Purveyors of hemp products sought to distinguish their non-narcotic textiles from the officially poisonous (or at least intoxicating) cannabis flower. The biggest push came in 1916, when the United States Department of Agriculture issued Bulletin No. 404, which concluded that paper created from hemp pulp was "favorable in comparison with those used with pulp wood" and that one acre of hemp would produce as much paper-ready pulp as four acres of trees. When the USDA's findings failed to revolutionize the paper manufacturing industry, hemp's most passionate supporters got suspicious, with the leading theory claiming that two American bigwigs—publisher William Randolph Hearst and the DuPont Corporation—conspired against hemp to protect their own paper-pulp interests. While this theory sounds reasonable, it's apparently bunk, with the main reason for hemp's limited success as an American textile being later studies that determined only one-third of the hemp stem produces durable fiber, securing hemp's stature as a semi-exotic textile.

While hemp foundered, recreational cannabis continued to gain favor throughout the early twentieth century.

Prohibition, paradoxically, helped; by outlawing alcohol, it led to a black market of costlier, harder-to-get bootleg booze, normalizing experimentation with also-illegal marijuana. First popularized among Mexican immigrants in the southwestern United States and jazz musicians in New Orleans and New York, marijuana soon found its way into popular culture. In Paramount Pictures' comedy spectacular of 1933 *International House,* Cab Calloway performed "Reefer Man," a song about a fellow whose love of marijuana makes him "trade dimes for nickels and call watermelon pickles."

Beyond poor money-management and fruit-identification skills, marijuana users were soon assumed to have many worse traits, thanks to the work of US government official Harry Anslinger. In 1930, he was picked to lead the new Federal Bureau of Narcotics, and immediately set about demonizing weed with the inflammatory melodrama of a Depression-era Nancy Grace. From impromptu axe murder to the reckless impregnation of America's daughters, the side effects Anslinger was ready to ascribe to marijuana seemed limited only by his

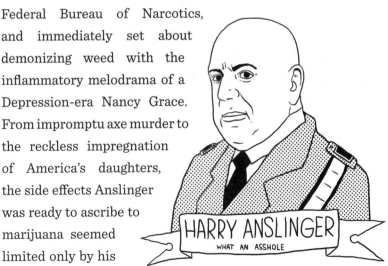

imagination and appetite for racist conjecture. (See Has Racism Played a Role in US Marijuana Laws? on the opposite page.)

In 1937, US lawmakers passed the Marihuana Tax Act, drafted by Anslinger and effectively making possession or transfer of cannabis illegal. Over objections from the American Medical Association, the legislation brought the end of over-the-counter cannabis medications, and in 1942, marijuana lost its last vestige of medical legitimacy when it was removed from US pharmacopeia.

The next several decades brought a back-and-forth battle between those who viewed marijuana as a minimally harmful intoxicant and helpful medicine, and those who wanted marijuana treated like a deadly poison.

New York City Mayor Fiorello LaGuardia directed the New York Academy of Medicine to investigate marijuana in 1938, with the ensuing report—1944's "The Marihuana Problem in the City of New York"—revealing key claims of scaremongers to be unfounded. Specifically, the LaGuardia Report found that smoking marijuana doesn't cause physical addiction, doesn't lead to use of harder narcotics, and isn't a determining factor in the commission of major crimes. "The publicity concerning the catastrophic effects of marijuana smoking in New York City is unfounded," stated the report.

Nevertheless, in 1951, the US Congress exploited the discredited "weed leads to heroin" myth to pass the Boggs

HAS RACISM PLAYED A ROLE IN
US MARIJUANA LAWS?

Dear God yes. The primary reason cannabis came to be perceived as a dangerous drug is that its use was first noted among those perceived to be dangerous people. "There are one hundred thousand total marijuana smokers in the US, and most are Negroes, Hispanics, Filipinos, and entertainers," said Federal Bureau of Narcotics chief Harry Anslinger in 1930. "Their Satanic music, jazz and swing result from marijuana use. This marijuana causes white women to seek sexual relations with Negroes, entertainers, and any others. . . . Reefer makes darkies think they're as good as white men." From these reprehensible roots grew the United States' current anti-marijuana legislation, which avoids Anslinger's rank bigotry while remaining effectively racist. In America, whites and blacks have all but equal rates of marijuana usage, but blacks are almost four times as likely to face a marijuana-related arrest. If US marijuana laws continue to be revised without commensurate revision of sentencing guidelines (including amnesty for sentencing victims), then we the people remain complicit in the same racist bullshit propagated by Harry Anslinger.

Act, a woeful bit of legislation that introduced mandatory sentencing to US law and made first-offense marijuana possession punishable with a minimum of two to ten years in prison and a fine of up to twenty thousand dollars.

This clash between scientific findings and the law characterized cannabis culture for most of the twentieth century. In 1968, the United Kingdom issued the Wootton Report, in which government scientists found that "cannabis in moderate doses has no harmful effects" and is safer than similar use of opiates, barbiturates, amphetamines, and alcohol. But the formative battle, with the furthest-reaching toxic effects commenced two years later in the United States, when Congress passed the Controlled Substances Act in 1970, which temporarily classified marijuana as a Schedule 1 drug, a designation reserved for intoxicants with the highest potential for abuse and no accepted medical use. However, before Congress was willing to saddle weed with a permanent Schedule 1 designation, it called for further research into the drug's effects and alleged dangers.

What followed was the National Commission on Marihuana and Drug Abuse, the most comprehensive weed study ever conducted by the US government, led by a team of congressmen, scientists, and law enforcement officials handpicked by President Richard Nixon, who was eager to have his grandstanding against the evils of weed supported by science. After a deep dive into all existing evidence, the

WILL MARIJUANA RENDER ME
CRIMINALLY INSANE AND KILL ME?

Probably not, but no one can blame you for being wary. For millennia, marijuana has been accused of arousing all sorts of harrowing states in users. In the greatest work of marijuana scaremongering, the 1936 film *Reefer Madness*, weed is presented as an all-purpose evil, inspiring users to commit rapes and murders en route to lifelong commitments in mental hospitals. Such cartoonishly monstrous depictions of marijuana use held sway in society until enough Americans had experienced weed's mellow pleasures for themselves. By the early 1970s, *Reefer Madness* was playing as a comedy on the midnight-movie circuit, and by the '80s, the old ploy of lumping cannabis with the hardest of hard drugs was no longer acceptable. The worst thing President Reagan's "War on Drugs" propaganda machine could say about marijuana is that it shouldn't be used by minors, drivers, and on-the-job surgeons. In the twenty-first century, the scariest stories being told about weed—that chronic use can damage memory, and that early chronic use might trigger mental illness—are all pretty much factual. Progress!

commission issued its report, which found that—surprise!—marijuana use did not lead to use of harder drugs, caused no significant damage to mind or body, and should be considered for legalization. "Marihuana's relative potential for harm to the vast majority of individual users and its actual impact on society does not justify a social policy designed to seek out and firmly punish those who use it," read the commission's report—to the violent dismay of President Nixon, an intractable weed hater who believed marijuana to be a cornerstone of a Jewish communist plot to overthrow the nation. (Seriously. He said as much on tape.) Whatever the case, Nixon publicly denounced his own commission's report and dismissed its findings, leaving marijuana stranded among Schedule 1 drugs, where it remains to this day.

A blow for sanity was struck in 1970, with the creation of the National Organization for the Reform of Marijuana Laws (NORML), a nonprofit, member-funded advocacy group devoted to ending marijuana prohibition in the United States. In 1972, NORML petitioned the Drug Enforcement Agency (DEA) to reschedule marijuana from Schedule 1 (designating drugs with no legitimate medical use that are unavailable in any legal way) to Schedule 2 (designating drugs with some medical use and available by prescription). After twenty-two years of federal foot-dragging, two direct orders to stop dallying from the US Court of Appeals, several futile attempts to solve the rescheduling debate through legislation, and a seemingly endless stream of conflicting testimony, the petition to reschedule cannabis was conclusively rejected in 1994, with the DEA Administrator citing the lack of verifiable scientific research on marijuana's medical benefits. (Fun fact: During the decades the DEA spent wrangling with the NORML petition, over thirty states passed laws recognizing the medical potential of marijuana.)

A small ray of hope arrived in 1980, when the National Cancer Institute began testing dronabinol, a synthetic form of THC taken orally in capsules, which in 1985 received FDA approval under the name Marinol. Initially sanctioned as a treatment for cancer patients experiencing nausea and vomiting during chemotherapy, Marinol was approved soon after for use as an antiemetic and appetite enhancer for people with AIDS and anorexia.

But things got awful on an exponential scale in 1986, with the Anti-Drug Abuse Act, a pernicious bit of "War on Drugs" legislation that, among other things, created new mandatory minimum sentences for marijuana-related offenses. The results were stark and terrifying. After ten years, federal prison populations had tripled, with one prisoner in six locked up on a marijuana offense, and those convicted of nonviolent marijuana charges sometimes serving longer than convicted murderers.

As federal prisons filled up with weed bustees, states got serious about protecting medical marijuana users.

WHICH PRESIDENTS WERE POTHEADS?
(AND VICE VERSA?)

The list of US presidents who experimented with marijuana ranges from rumored users to confessed aficionados. Among the rumored are two Founding Fathers—George Washington and Thomas Jefferson, both of whom grew hemp on their plantations and have since been saddled with all sorts of presidential pothead lore. In truth, there's no proof either Washington or Jefferson ever imbibed THC, which makes the first president to definitely have used the products of the hemp plant to achieve psychotropic effect James Monroe, POTUS #5, who openly smoked hashish while serving as ambassador to France. The mid-nineteenth century brought a sudden rush of THC into presidential bloodstreams, as both Zachary Taylor (president #12) and Franklin Pierce (president #14) were military men who recounted smoking marijuana with the troops while fighting the Mexican-American War. In the twentieth century, use by future presidents grew: John F. Kennedy reportedly used marijuana to allay severe back pain, and both Bill Clinton and George W. Bush copped to experimenting with recreational marijuana, with the fork-tongued Clinton qualifying his confession by saying he "didn't inhale." "I inhaled, frequently," said Barack Obama about his teenage weed use. "That was the point." Beyond the zingy quip, Obama made good on his promise as America's most pro-pot president, taking steps to dismantle some of the grosser excesses of Reagan's "War on Drugs" legislation and instructing federal prosecutors to stop pursuing medical marijuana users in states where such use is legal.

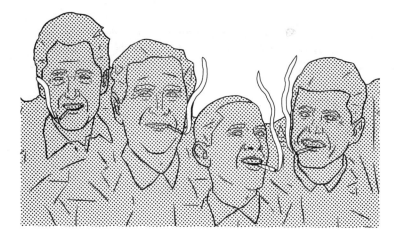

California led the charge, legalizing cannabis for authorized patients in 1996. Alaska, Oregon, Washington, and Maine soon followed suit, and over the next two decades, twenty-three states would enact laws protecting the medical use of marijuana. (Meanwhile, Canada proactively skipped the roll-out and became the first country on earth to approve medical marijuana nationwide in 2003.)

As for recreational weed: The twenty-first century continued the upswing in usage charted since 1977, when 24 percent of Americans reported having tried marijuana at least once in their lives. By 2013, that number was up to 38 percent, with eighteen million Americans—7 percent of the population aged twelve and up—reporting using weed within the past month.

NOTABLE MOMENTS IN MARIJUANA HISTORY

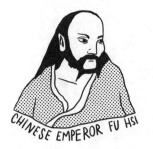

FU HSI: 2900 BCE

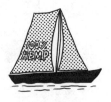

HEMP SAIL: 1533

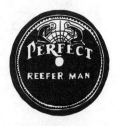

REEFER MAN
RECORD: 1933

To accommodate recreational weed's growing grass-roots popularity, US cities began taking baby steps toward decriminalization: if they couldn't just legalize it, they could at least downgrade its vilification. By 2013, sixteen cities passed ordinances requiring police to treat non-disruptive weed possession by adults as the "lowest law-enforcement priority."

Massachusetts jump-started the movement for full-on decriminalization on a state level in 2008, when voters turned simple possession of up to one ounce of marijuana from a criminal offense punishable by jail to a civil infraction punishable by a hundred dollar fine. In 2011, Connecticut also decriminalized the possession of small amounts of cannabis, and in 2012, Washington and Colorado took the full plunge, becoming the first states in the nation to officially

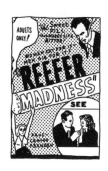

REEFER MADNESS: 1936

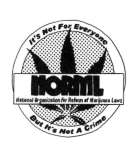

NORML: 1970

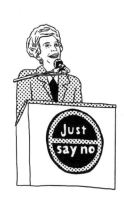

JUST SAY NO: 1986

legalize the recreational use of cannabis in state law. In 2014, Alaska, Oregon, and Washington, DC, joined them, and it's easy to imagine other states will soon follow suit. (One reason they probably will: the first year of legal weed in Colorado generated seven hundred million dollars in business, created sixty-three million in tax revenue, and collected an additional thirteen million in licenses and fees, and America loves giant piles of money.)

What's next for weed? Answers are gathering all around us in the form of legislative pushes for revision of marijuana laws and sentencing guidelines, plus legalization of medically beneficial low-THC weed. Add to this a populace that's increasingly unwilling to accept the government's lies about weed's dangers and ignorance of its benefits, and the United States could finally become a nation where marijuana's medicinal properties are fully harnessed, and where weed takes its rightful place alongside alcohol on the shelf of legal American intoxicants.

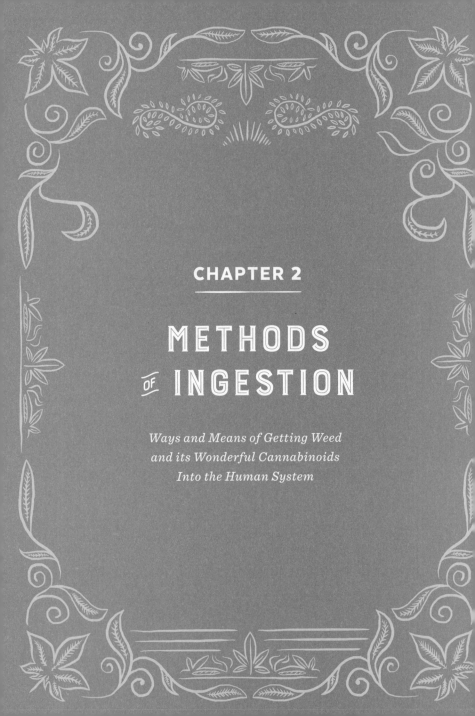

CHAPTER 2

METHODS of INGESTION

*Ways and Means of Getting Weed
and its Wonderful Cannabinoids
Into the Human System*

From hand-rolled cigarettes to THC-infused food to creatively deployed hot plates, the tools and methods for escorting weed into the human system are multitudinous. But things break down into three basic camps: **inhalation** (of smoke or vapor), **oral ingestion** (of THC-infused food, drink, or capsules), and **topical application** (stuff you rub on your skin). Each has its own benefits, hindrances, and specific effects. Shall we?

INHALATION

Whether you're dealing with smoke from a bong or mist from a vaporizer, the basic high-making principles of inhaled THC remain the same. Cannabinoids are drawn into the lungs and escorted via alveoli into the bloodstream, where they immediately begin binding with receptors throughout the brain and the rest of the nervous system. Easily the quickest method of getting high, smoking/vaping produces noticeable effects within two to three minutes and a high that lasts between two and three hours. (Inhalation is a good method for the THC novice—the quick onset of effects makes it harder to accidentally get too high, and the relatively short duration of the high will be a comfort for those who don't like it.)

﹌ JOINTS ﹏
a.k.a. marijuana cigarettes

This is a no-frills classic. Joints work best not with sticky-icky bud, but with drier chunks of weed, which should be broken down into flakey, fluffy bits before being rolled. Helpful tools: a grinder (a small, handheld device that breaks marijuana buds down into perfect soft flakes) and a cigarette-rolling machine, both of which are available for cheap at any tobacco store. To learn how to roll a joint, see pages 83 to 92.

﹌ BLUNTS ﹏

Blunts are joints rolled not with cigarette rolling papers but with cigar papers, which are made of tobacco leaf. The result is a slower-burning joint that delivers an extra blast of nicotine—a crucial fact for blunt lovers who appreciate the THC/tobacco combo, and a deterrent to those wary of combining minimally addictive THC with seriously addictive nicotine.

﹌ SPLIFFS ﹏

Spliffs are joints made with regular rolling papers filled with a mix of marijuana and tobacco. Spliff lovers tout the weed-conserving habit of joints that are half tobacco, and say the nicotine extends the duration of the effects of the THC. Spliff doubters don't want to muck up their highs or personal narratives by smoking tobacco.

JOINTS

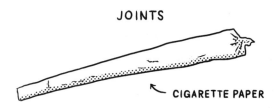

CIGARETTE PAPER

BLUNTS

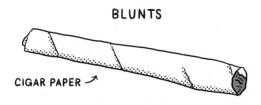

CIGAR PAPER

SPLIFFS

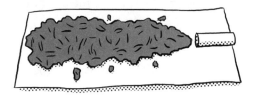

A MIX OF WEED AND TOBACCO

৶ PIPES ৶

Even easier to use than joints (no rolling, just stuffing-and-puffing!), pipes involve a bowl, a suction chamber, and a mouthpiece, all of which come in an ever-expanding variety of shapes and sizes. But the key factor is material.

✹ **METAL PIPES** are small, inexpensive, and indestructible, and thus great for on-the-go smoking. Unfortunately, metal heats up fast, quickly turning a pass-the-pipe situation involving more than two people into a lip-and-finger torture session.

✹ **WOODEN PIPES** are slightly more expensive than metal options but are prettier and more user friendly. (They only become too hot to handle if they're actually on fire.) Small wooden pipes are great for on the go, but larger ones bestow a certain Gandalfiness and are best kept at home.

✹ **GLASS AND CERAMIC PIPES** are a pricier option, but they can be pretty and feel more like cherished objects than disposable tools. They are great for home use but too fragile for on the go. (Glass pipes are plenty sturdy, but one drop on a sidewalk and smashboohoo.)

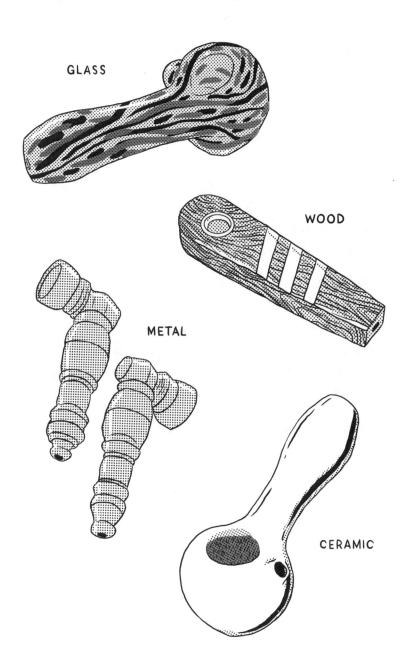

GLASS

WOOD

METAL

CERAMIC

⚹ **ONE-HITTERS** are small cylindrical metal pipes that function like cigarettes, with a "bowl," a little hole that runs in a direct line to the mouthpiece. The compactness of the bowl hole makes an appropriately tight container to keep your weed from falling out—hold a one-hitter more or less parallel to the ground and you're set. However, one-hitters are screenless, making it easy for overzealous users to suck bits of burning weed or ash into their mouths. This is exactly as fun as it sounds. Draw lightly. (For more on pipe screens, see To Screen or Not to Screen? on page 32.)

⚹ Speaking of one-hitters, **DUGOUTS** are small, dual-chambered containers that hold a small amount of weed in one chamber and a one-hitter pipe in the other. To load a bowl, the open mouth of the pipe is pressed down into the weed chamber and lightly twisted, which perfectly packs the bowl.

⚹ Meanwhile, **STOGIES** function just like one-hitters, but rather than a millimeters-wide bowl, a stogie's bowl spans a half inch—big enough to hold a sizey bud *and* accept a screen, thus sidestepping the skimpy servings and ashy-mouthed troubles of the basic one-hitter. This fat-mouthed bowl is attached to a stubby metal pipe, which is fitted at the suction end with a rubber mouthpiece to keep lips from sizzling on the fast-heating metal. At the bowl end is a screw-on cover with a tiny smoke hole, allowing a flame to enter while safely containing the weed—an exemplary method of stealth on-the-go smoking.

★ Finally, **DISGUISE PIPES** are gimmicky plastic creations that hide a functional pipe within an eye-tricking disguise. One popular option looks like a standard chubby highlighter marker, until you unscrew the parts to reveal a bowl and mouthpiece. Unfortunately, smoking from such a device involves the close proximity of fire and plastic, which is unappealing for all sorts of commonsense chemical reasons. This is why disguise pipes are typically used only as a last resort. (A notable exception: metal one-hitters designed to look like cigarettes, which involve zero plastic and are great camouflage.)

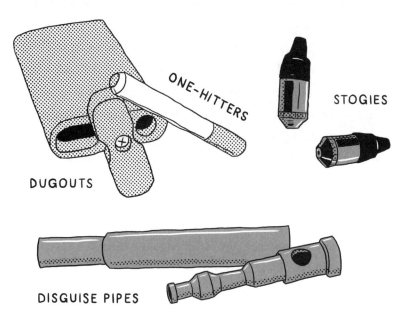

ONE-HITTERS

STOGIES

DUGOUTS

DISGUISE PIPES

৬ WATER PIPES ৬
a.k.a. bongs, bubblers

A water pipe is a larger, non-portable device in which the basic pipe components—bowl, suction chamber, mouthpiece—are enhanced with water, which is added to the pipe's expanded suction chamber. As the user inhales, smoke passes through the water before entering the user's mouth and lungs, making for a cooler, smoother smoking experience.

Bongs are beloved by weed smokers for the cooler-and-smoother thing mentioned above, and also for their oversize suction chambers, which allow users to ingest a large mass of weed smoke in a smooth single inhalation. Key to the bong's process: the carburetion port, or "carb," a small hole placed in a conspicuous spot along the suction chamber. During inhalation, the carb hole is covered with a thumb or finger to allow the inhaled smoke to fill the length of the chamber—after which the thumb or finger is moved, the carb hole is exposed, and air rushes into the chamber and sends the gathered smoke racing into a user's lungs. (Some bongs are rigged not with a hole but with what's called "pull carb," wherein air is let into the chamber by lifting the airtight bowl from its stem. For full information, see How to Use a Bong on page 97.)

If bong hits sound vaguely aggressive, you're not wrong. Still, a small, sensible puff off a bong—letting the chamber fill with a wisp of smoke rather than a dense fog—is a delightful way to get a quick, strong high. (But if you're a newbie or casual user, you should still probably aim to take your small, sensible puff off a joint or pipe or vaporizer—by design, big-chambered bongs are more for serious users.)

🌿 **PLASTIC BONGS** are cheap, light, durable, and get the job done.

🌿 **GLASS BONGS** are pricier, prettier, simultaneously heavier and more fragile, and generally superior to plastic bongs. Glass bongs come in an array of artsy designs and are the easiest bongs to keep clean.

🌿 **CERAMIC BONGS** take the creativity to another level, with water pipes shaped like penises or squatting wizards. When choosing a bong, one question should rank above all others: How easy will this bong be to clean? Unfortunately, kooky shapes can seriously impede cleaning, and for the hygienic bong huffer, all roads lead to a straight glass tube.

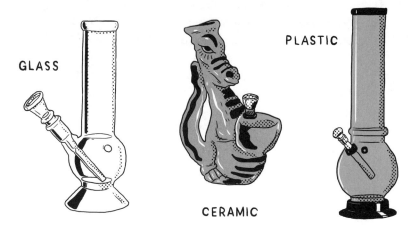

GLASS

PLASTIC

CERAMIC

TO SCREEN OR NOT TO SCREEN?

Pipe screens are—surprise!—screens placed in pipes to keep the sucked-upon burning material from entering the mouths of suckers. Screens come in an array of sizes (quarter- and half-inch are the most common) and are typically made of brass or stainless steel. If your weed is in large dense buds—which naturally bind together as they burn—you may not need a screen. But when dealing with smaller, finer bits of weed, all smoking devices benefit from a screen, which is shoved down into a pipe/bong's bowl with the aim of covering the suction hole.

Using a screen in a glass pipe can be tricky, as a clean glass bowl is a shallow, slippery thing that requires your screen to balance precariously over the bowl hole. However, a couple dozen puffs on a clean bowl will soon render it a slightly dirty bowl, laced with a sticky resin that is incredibly helpful in keeping a screen in place. If your glass pipe has a deeper bowl, consider bending the screen with your finger or a pen cap to better fit the bowl's shape.

In addition to the aforementioned steel and brass options, there is a third screen type: glass, sometimes called glass gauzes or glass jacks. Available for cheap at tobacco shops, these glass devices rest at the *bottom* of a bong's bowl to block material from being sucked into the body of the bong.

If you're using a bong, all the basic rules apply: unless you're using super-sticky bud that binds together as it burns, you'll want to use a screen.

✶ Essentially the love child of a pipe and a bong, a **BUBBLER** is a glass or ceramic pipe that incorporates a water chamber and a carb, affording users cool smoke and a sensibly downsized bong-like experience.

✶ Originating in Persia, the **HOOKAH** is a luxurious water pipe outfitted with a large bowl and numerous individual suction tubes, which are deployed like octopus arms and allow for simultaneous communal smoking. Smoking weed in a hookah can be done bong-style, where a screen is placed in the hookah's bowl and the weed is ignited with a lighter, or traditional hookah style, where weed is mixed with shisha tobacco and leisurely burnt over charcoal. Why don't weed smokers use hookahs all the time? Mostly because hookahs burn a lot of weed, waste a lot of smoke, and are a pain in the butt to clean. (Imagine cleaning the insides of a half-dozen bendy bong chambers attached like snakes to Medusa's head.)

✑ FUNKY HOMEMADE DEVICES ✑

When there is marijuana to smoke, but no paper or pipe in which to smoke it, humans get creative.

✶ **HOT KNIVES** are a crude kitchen classic, involving two metal butter knives heated on a stove burner or electric hot plate until the knives' tips are dangerously hot, after which a small bit of weed or hash is placed onto one burning knife tip, compressed with the other burning knife tip, and abruptly turned into a blast of super-dense smoke, which is inhaled through a funnel (typically an empty paper-towel roll) into the user's mouth. If this sounds complicated, dangerous, and borderline stupid, you're right—but it's the best way to make a teeny bit of weed pack a big punch, and so will remain part of the young and/or occasionally desperate smoker's arsenal. If hot knives sound like something you want to try, make sure your fire insurance premiums are paid and buy cheap metal knives from Goodwill, as no knife used for hot-knifing can ever be used for anything else again.

🌿 If there's a method of weed smoking that screams "I am young and dumb" louder than hot knives, it's the **GRAVITY BONG**, an even more complicated method of smoke inhalation involving a bucket of water, a two-liter plastic bottle cut in half and rigged with a smoking bowl, and strategically deployed air pressure that literally forces smoke into a user's lungs. Perfect for those who want to get alarmingly high without having to do the hard work of inhaling, gravity bongs are essentially the keg stands of the weed world—a party trick for less-than-mature partiers that's way more trouble than it's worth. (If you insist on trying a gravity bong at least once, you can find instructions on how to make one on the Internet.)

🌿 A similar "reckless adolescent" vibe hovers around the **ALUMINUM CAN PIPE**, a brutally simple device that involves denting a "bowl" in the side of an empty aluminum can, stabbing a collection of small smoke holes around the bottom of the bowl, and inhaling through the mouth hole. If you're ever trapped in a hotel with only weed and a soda machine, a can pipe can be a lifesaver.

🌿 On the healthier side, an **APPLE** can be turned into a makeshift pipe in a manner similar to a can, but with less violence and fewer worries about inhaling whatever chemicals might be released from a burning aluminum can. For the full story, see How to Turn an Apple into a Pipe on page 95.

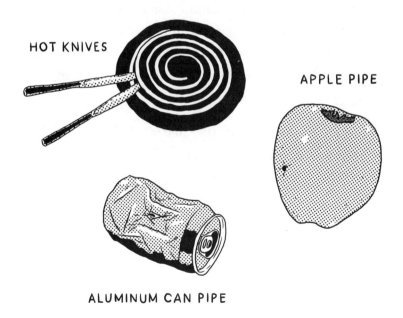

HOT KNIVES

APPLE PIPE

ALUMINUM CAN PIPE

⌇ VAPORIZERS ⌇

A single-handed fix for many unwelcome aspects of smoking weed, a vaporizer heats marijuana to a temperature high enough to release cannabinoids but low enough to avoid combustion. This gives users all the pleasures of smoking with no gross by-products of burning like carbon monoxide and tar. What's released from heated-not-burnt weed is a vapor with the faint smell of yesterday's popcorn. It's a world away from the room-filling skunk fog of smoked weed. Much cooler in temperature than smoke, weed vapor is naturally more gentle on throats and lungs, and has been found to have a slightly higher THC concentration than pot smoke. If that's not enough, vaporizing is a significantly more efficient method of extracting cannabinoids from weed, with vapor inhalers alleging that half as much weed will get you twice as high.

A NOTE ABOUT SMOKING

Fact: Inhaling smoke from burning material is not good for humans. Smoking marijuana involves inhaling thousands of chemicals, one of which is the point-of-it-all high-making compound THC, while many others are known carcinogens, which are present at higher levels than in unfiltered tobacco smoke. Not helping is the habit of weed smokers to inhale deeply and hold smoke in for an extended time, resulting in elevated levels of carbon monoxide and tar in their lungs.

Does the inhalation of all these weedy carcinogens have a track record of adding up to cancer? Weirdly, no. Historically, studies of the connection between marijuana smoking and cancer risk have been complicated by subjects' simultaneous smoking of highly carcinogenic tobacco, but 2013 brought a study of marijuana-only smokers, and the worst thing found was some tissue alteration recognized as a precursor to the development of cancer in the lungs of the heaviest smokers. But for light and moderate weed smokers, studies have found no increased risk of lung or upper-airway cancers. Unlike cigarettes, smoking weed has no link to pulmonary disease, reduced lung function, or respiratory tract infections. Most surprisingly, recent studies have suggested marijuana actually *decreases* the risk of lung cancer (?!), with recent cell and animal studies confirming marijuana's ability to kill cancer cells (!!). For more on the intersection of marijuana and cancer, see Chapter 9: Medical Marijuana 101.

Even with cancer a downgraded risk, there are still plenty of downsides to smoking, from hacking coughs to smelly houses. But what's crucial to remember is that **marijuana itself is not carcinogenic**—only when weed is burned and inhaled do carcinogens and respiratory irritants come into play. Lucky for all, there's an ever-expanding universe of options for smoke-free weed, beginning with vaporizers (see opposite page).

Considering these benefits, perhaps you're wondering why the nation's Dumpsters aren't overflowing with bongs, as all humanity turns to the superior pleasures of vaping.

One explanation: some people love to smoke weed and cherish the exact components of smoking that repel others, from the burning smoke and befouled air to the eye-bulging coughing fits. For such folks, the subtler delivery system of the vaporizer just can't compete with being punched in the lungs by burning bong smoke. But if you're a new user, I hereby order you to run toward a vaporizer and never look back. (And confidential to bong-trained pot smokers: a full bag of dense vapor from the top-of-the-line Volcano vaporizer is reportedly vaping's best approximation of a good old-fashioned bong hit.)

★ **DESKTOP VAPORIZERS** plug into the wall for use at home. Such "fixed models" are typically made of metal and/or glass and range in price from $99 to $420. This is how they work: weed is placed is the extraction chamber, the internal heating element is activated, and for the next few minutes the weed slowly and steadily releases cannabinoids in a vapor that is either inhaled directly through a hose or collected in an inflatable plastic bag and inhaled soon after. (Keeping vapor in a bag for any length of time is unwise. Puffing on a bag of vapor over a few minutes is fine, but extended storage can result in significant loss of THC.) Deluxe desktop vaporizers offer temperature control, which allows users to target specific cannabinoids to attain a particular type of high. For example, lower vaporizing temperatures reportedly activate cannabinoids that result in a more energetic "daytime high," while higher temperatures create a more body-centric, sedative "nighttime high."

HOW MUCH WEED SHOULD I SMOKE TO GET HIGH?

One great thing about smoking weed is that the effects land within minutes, so the best way to answer the question "How much weed should I smoke to get high?" is to take a puff or two, wait five minutes, and see how you feel. If after five minutes you're not as high as you'd like, repeat until satisfied. The main thing to remember is to start slow. It's very easy to get more high, and very hard to get less high, so ramp up in increments and don't follow anyone's lead but your own. (Veteran smokers can take fifty bong hits and seem perfectly normal, while novices can be laid out by a puff and a half off a joint.)

★ Compressing the whole extraction chamber/heating element situation into a simple pocket-size device, **PORTABLE VAPORIZERS** are hands down the best method for getting high without getting noticed. Portable vaporizers range from thirty-dollar-and-up e-cigarette-type "vape pens" to small, state-of-the-art pocket vapor factories that run upward of two hundred fifty dollars. Some portable vaporizers accept weed, others use cartridges of smokable oils, and some work with both. No matter what you're vaping, what's released is that same popcorny barely-a-smell, enabling vapers to do their thing pretty much anywhere they want.

✹ A newfangled version of hot knives (see page 33), **DABBING** is a form of vaporization in which freakishly potent cannabis concentrates (hash oil, shatter, "wax") are placed on a small metal surface that's been heated with a blowtorch, creating a dense blast of vapor that some have likened to "snorting a line of cannabinoids." Dabbing is undoubtedly effective—even people who get high all day, every day, will be made extraordinarily high by a good dab. But it's pretty much an elite sport for heavy users. (For more on shatter and other cannabis concentrates, see Beyond Weed on page 55.)

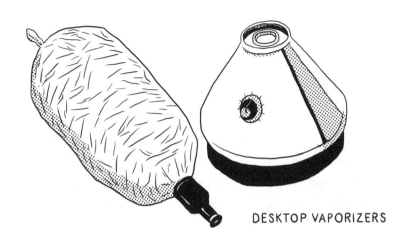

DESKTOP VAPORIZERS

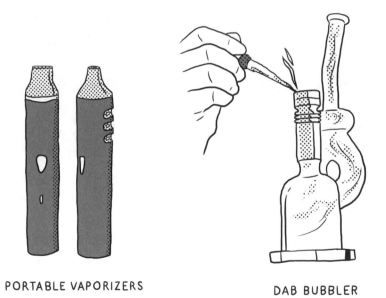

PORTABLE VAPORIZERS

DAB BUBBLER

ORAL INGESTION
a.k.a. eatin' 'n' drinkin'

Beyond smoking and vaping exists a world of cannabis consumption that avoids inhalation entirely, bypassing the lungs for the stomach. The variety of cannabis-enhanced edibles—cookies, brownies, candy, soda, Chex Mix, spaghetti sauce—is huge and expanding daily. Before we start parsing the menu, here are some basic facts.

Eating cannabis-enhanced food or drink offers an experience that is so distinct from smoking weed that edible marijuana should be considered a different drug—just because you enjoy smoking cannabis doesn't mean you'll enjoy eating it, and vice versa.

The first key difference is in how orally ingested cannabinoids enter the user's system. Whereas smoked/vaporized weed races into the bloodstream via the lungs, eaten weed enters the system much more slowly, progressing from the stomach to the liver—which transforms basic THC into stronger 11-hydroxy-THC—before entering the bloodstream. Extended along with the wait time is the high's duration—the effects from orally ingested weed take between one and two hours to hit, after which the high will last between five and nine hours. I repeat: THE HIGH WILL LAST BETWEEN

FIVE AND NINE HOURS. This is a very different proposition than a puff or vape, where the high hits in minutes and dissipates in the time it takes to watch *Die Hard*. Edibles deliver a bone-deep body high, which hits and sticks and can sometimes feel lightly narcotic and even hallucinogenic.

If you are someone who does not want to be narcotically high for five-plus hours, you should steer clear of edible marijuana. If you're a curious new user—especially a newbie visiting a post-prohibition city like Denver or Seattle, where delectable, industrial-grade weed treats abound—please read the following carefully.

⨳ EDIBLES ⨳

Getting high from eating marijuana doesn't mean just shoving weed in your mouth and chewing (which gets you nothing but wasted pot and weed-flecked teeth). Cannabinoids are lipophilic—activated when dissolved in lipids—and for edible marijuana to bestow a high, the cannabinoids must be drawn out of the weed with a solvent fat such as butter or olive oil. This cannabinoid-enhanced butter or oil is then used in recipes and food prep just like regular butter and oil.

Take, for example, the iconic pot brownie. With brownies, as in most weed-enhanced baked goods (fudge, cookies, "space cakes"), the cannabinoids come along with the butter, and literally anything that can be made with butter—from pancakes to baked potatoes—can be enhanced with cannabinoids.

Cannabinoids can also be drawn out of weed with olive and vegetable oils, which opens up a world beyond dessert and into savory options. As with butter, enhanced oil can be used in any recipe that calls for non-enhanced oil—for more information, see the recipe for Cannabis-Infused Cooking Oil on page 75.

Another wonderful edible option available in post-prohibition/pro-medical marijuana states involves no butter or cooking oil, just highly concentrated hash oil, which is injected into everything from gummy bears to energy drinks, giving users serious, long-lasting highs.

Clearly there are many reasons to love edible marijuana: the extended effects, the bypassing of smoking, the ease and stealth of consumption. (Weed cookies look just like normal cookies!) But there are also distinct drawbacks, including empty calories from sugar and fat, and certain items' visual appeal to children. (Weed cookies look just like normal cookies!) But the primary drawback of edible weed involves the aforementioned extended duration of both the pre-high wait time and the high itself, two really, really important considerations that demand their own section.

THE PERILS OF EDIBLES, OR HOW TO EAT
WEED WITHOUT WANTING TO BE DEAD

For all its pleasures, edible marijuana is fraught with hazards, and these hazards can be strangely counterintuitive. Take weed-enhanced cookies and candy—with their appealing and familiar shapes, they seem like the perfect training-wheel version of weed. Certainly a bong hit is a more serious business than eating a cookie, right? But the opposite is true: edible weed, no matter how homey the delivery method, bestows a deeper, longer, stronger high than the gnarliest bong rip.

Further complications can arise from expectations regarding serving size. In the regular world, a candy bar or a cookie is considered "a serving." But in the world of professionally made marijuana edibles, one enhanced candy bar or cookie can contain multiple doses of weed. Such dosage specifics are printed on the product's packaging, but the human drive to eat all of a cookie is strong, so even with explicit labeling, users still might be confused about exactly how many milligrams of THC add up to a representative serving. (Five to ten milligrams of THC equals roughly one serving for a newbie, FYI.) Homemade edibles can be even trickier, as the butter-based cannabinoid delivery system can spread the THC over a whole batch of a baked good, making one brownie in the batch weaker and another stronger, and good luck guessing which is which.

But the riskiest factor is the slow onset of effects, which tempts impatient users to deduce that "it's not working" or they "didn't take enough," two phrases that regularly land weed eaters in the paralyzing swamp of over-highness that threatened to devour *New York Times* columnist Maureen Dowd, who traveled to Colorado, ate too much of an THC-enhanced candy bar, and wrote a column about the now-infamous nightmare that followed.

So what does a weed eater need to avoid such a fate? **Patience**, which isn't something naturally associated with the escapist pleasures of getting high but is absolutely mandatory for proper enjoyment of edible marijuana. Along with patience, there are a few simple rules weed eaters need to adhere to:

✴ **DECIDE ON DOSAGE.** Five to ten milligrams of THC is the recommended "single serving" for new users, while seasoned users will find perfectly comfortable highs with thirty to fifty milligrams and up.

✴ Whatever your dosage, once you ingest it you should **WRITE DOWN THE TIME** and remind yourself that you are forbidden to even consider ingesting more weed-enhanced anything for at least two hours. Set a timer.

✴ **RELAX AND WAIT** for your high to hit. For most users, effects land within forty-five minutes to an hour. For others, especially new users, effects may not land for up to two hours. This is the reason for the **mandatory two-hour wait time** between one dose of edible THC and another. Few supposedly fun things are suckier than an accidental weed overdose, which can't actually hurt you (no one has ever died from too much weed), but can strand users in a strange and terrifying place for a few hours, which is no fun and so easy to avoid. If you're easily bored and given to impatience, use the movie method: immediately after eating a dose of edible marijuana, sit down and watch a movie. (May I suggest the perfect one hour and fifty-nine minutes that is *The Grifters*?) If you don't feel high by the movie's end, feel free to consider another dose. (And if you do indulge, the two-hour wait time starts over again.) Should you ever find yourself too high, don't wig out, just relax, and see Chapter 7: If You're High and Don't Like It.

EXPERIENCE LEVEL	DOSE
New to weed or returning after years of abstinence	Small dose (5 to 10 mg THC)
Smoke weed every once in a while	Intermediate dose (15 to 30 mg THC)
Smoke weed all the time	Veteran dose (30 to 50 mg THC)

✺ DRINKABLES ✺

Getting high by drinking THC isn't as simple as tossing weed in hot water and calling it tea. Because of cannabinoids' fat solubility, fat or another solvent is required to release the psychoactive effects. Historically, most marijuana beverages have been milk- or alcohol-based. However, thanks to more recent developments with cannabis concentrates, a new world of THC-infused beverages has opened up, bringing us tons of hash-oil-spiked sodas and juices and energy drinks. (Fun fact: They do not taste at all disgusting.) As with edibles, drinkable THC is ingested through the stomach and processed by the liver, so wait the minimum mandatory two hours between doses.

✺ TINCTURES ✺

A tincture is a marijuana concentrate in an alcohol solution, which is administered in liquid drops. Taken under the tongue, the THC-enhanced drops race into the bloodstream with the speed of smoke or vapor. Added to food or drink, the cannabinoids are processed more leisurely by the liver, mandating a two-hour wait time between doses.

Good things about a tincture: stealth, avoidance of smoke, and its non-deliciousness (which skirts the temptations of yummy weed treats). Less-good things about a tincture: It tastes gross, especially if you go with the under-the-tongue method, which floods your face with the taste of dirty bong water laced with tequila, thanks to the harsh alcohol base. But adding tincture drops to another, non-disgusting liquid (orange juice, chocolate milk, V-8) cuts the grossness almost entirely. For more, see Cannabis Tincture on page 80.

✒ CONCENTRATED OILS ✒

Concentrated cannabis oils are known by a variety of names—hash oil, honey oil, butane hash oil (BHO), shatter, wax—but they're all made in the same general way. Cannabinoids from marijuana are extracted in alcohol, which is then left to evaporate. What's left behind is a tar-like substance that can be smoked, vaped, or ingested orally, and will get you very high. Among the oral-ingestion offerings are hash-oil capsules and oil-infused candies (e.g., Cinnamon Bears, "Sour Pot Kids"). Among the smokable/vapable options are shatter, wax, and BHO, all of which can be ingested via pipe (where the hash-oil component typically rests atop a bed of regular weed), bong (ditto), vaporizer, or dabbing. Smoked/vaped oils hit immediately and keep users high for a couple hours, while orally ingested oils take up to two hours to hit and keep users high for six-plus hours (two-hour wait rule applies).

TOPICAL APPLICATIONS

If you'd like to leave your lungs and digestive system out of your marijuana experience, the world of cannabinoid-rich lotions, balms, and salves might be for you. Applied directly to your skin, the compounds of cannabis lotions penetrate no deeper than the muscles, where they can work wonders for joint diseases, muscle soreness, and skin conditions like psoriasis and eczema. But such topicals stop short of the bloodstream, rendering them non-psychoactive and thus worthless for high seekers.

However, more recent developments have brought topical applications capable of penetrating deeply enough to flood the bloodstream with cannabinoids and send users to happy high land. Such transdermal THC applications range from controlled-release patches to roll-on lotions, and as they bypass the digestive system and liver, deliver a high within minutes.

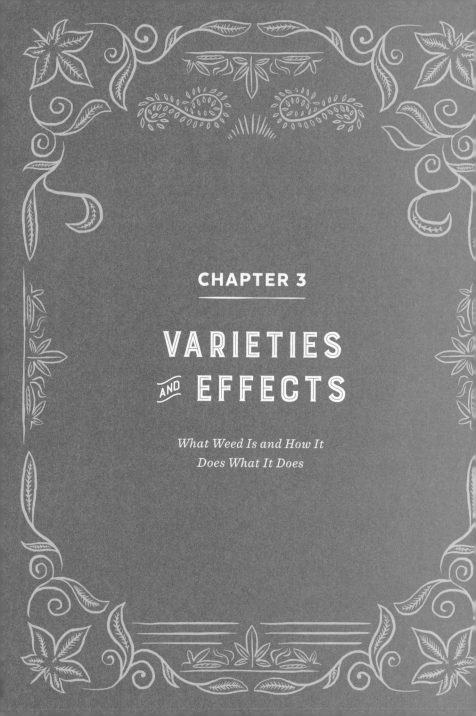

CHAPTER 3

VARIETIES AND EFFECTS

*What Weed Is and How It
Does What It Does*

F rom classics like Kush and Haze to new specialties like Strawberry Cough and Boggle Dragon, the variety of cannabis strains is vast and getting vaster, as growers target specific characteristics and effects, and legal-weed retailers aim for eye-catching products. (Why settle for Purple Haze when you can have Green Crack?) But underneath all the hilarious names lie two basic strains, *Cannabis sativa* and *Cannabis indica*, which form the key divide in the world of weed usage.

Sativa plants are tall, thin, narrow-leafed, and native to warm climates, where they're quick to grow but slow to flower. Sativas are known for producing a high that users describe as cerebral and energetic, conducive to creative labors and the enhancement of art and entertainment.

Indicas are short, bushy, wide-leafed plants native to Afghanistan, Morocco, and Tibet, where harsher climates speed up the flowering process and inspire the plant's development of a protective coat of resin, adding up to a high users describe as more of a sedative, body-based experience, conducive to sinking

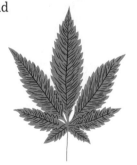

SATIVA

INDICA

into the couch while playing *Grand Theft Auto XVII* for five hours and then sleeping like a rock.

Fun fact: Despite their differences, sativa and indica are classified as the exact same plant (cannabis), in the same way that poodles and pit bulls are classified as the exact same species (canine). To carry this "strains equal breeds" comparison further, a sativa high is like a superintelligent terrier that cracks you up and inspires your poetry, while an indica high is a lazy sheepdog that pins you to the sofa until you feed it enough Doritos. (Metaphor not legally binding.)

However, some say such ironclad distinctions between sativa and indica are overstated, with the key differences between strains coming from **terpenes**, the aromatic oils contained in cannabis resin, which modulate and mingle with cannabinoids to produce singular effects. (The terpene **myrcene**, for example, enhances weed's psychoactive effects, while the terpene **terpinol** amps sedative effects.)

But the happy truth is that most cannabis strains available today are hybrids, blending indica and sativa (and their terpenes) in various measures to achieve various effects, and

---

TIMING TIPS

Sativa before bedtime is unwise for anyone with insomnia issues, and an a.m. indica blast can absorb a full day's worth of motivation. Aim accordingly.

---

the basic distinction between sativa and indica remains valuable, especially for those looking to avoid undesired effects.

BEYOND WEED: HASH, SHATTER, WAX, BHO, KIEF, 🖋️ THE WORLD OF THC CONCENTRATES

In THC concentrates, the cannabis flower is stripped of its pleasurable cannabinoids and processed into a variety of dense, sticky substances that, when smoked or vaporized, get users very high for a long time. **Hashish** is the ancient classic, in which the THC-rich trichomes that gather on marijuana flowers are separated from the plant, collected in a mass, and pressed into a firm, smokable clay-like substance. To make **wax**, THC is extracted from marijuana with butane, which evaporates to leave a goopy substance that resembles—surprise!—wax. **Shatter** involves not one but two butane extractions, to create a THC-drenched substance that's smooth, clear, and so hard it can shatter like glass. **BHO** is the abbreviation used for butane hash oil (sometimes called butane honey oil), yet another butane extraction that results in a viscous, resinous substance. And **kief** is the laid-back cousin of hashish, in which marijuana bud's trichomes are removed, collected, and left as unpressed flaky bits, to be added to joints and pipes.

As with marijuana flower, concentrates come as either sativa-dominant or indica-dominant, and all of the aforementioned products can be smoked via all the methods used for weed. (In pipes and bongs, hash products are typically placed on top of bowls filled with weed, while vaporizers do fine with just the straight-up hash product.)

Make no mistake, the point of all of the above concentrates is to pack a major THC wallop, making them a good fit for serious users who want to stay very high for a long time, and a not-so-good fit for casual users and beginners.

THC FEELINGS: AN OVERVIEW

The basic mechanics of getting high remain the same whether you're smoking weed, vaporizing hash, or scarfing a cannabutter croissant. Leading the charge and doing most of the heavy lifting: **cannabinoids**, the chemical compounds found in marijuana that act on receptors throughout our brains and bodies to produce the array of feelings known as being high. Scientists have identified eighty-five different cannabinoids, the most beloved and psychoactively powerful of which is tetrahydrocannabinol, hereby abbreviated to THC.

How it works: after passing through weed smokers' lungs (or weed-eaters' stomachs and livers), THC and its fellow cannabinoids ride the bloodstream to the brain, where they begin binding with receptors and disrupting transmission of neural signals. The first flush of highness comes with an increased heart rate that sends THC-enhanced blood rushing through the body, followed by a steadily accumulating array of effects associated with being high, from relaxation and euphoria to enhanced hunger and kaleidoscopic thinking.

IS WEED AN APHRODISIAC?

Technically speaking, no. Weed can do a great many things to enhance sex once it's happening, but it's not a sexual stimulant—it won't inspire sex, but it can inspire those interested in having sex to get super into it. Kissing, sucking, licking, touching, being touched—all these activities can become epic adventures in the slo-mo, sensory-enhanced world of weed. If you are someone who enjoys sex (by yourself or with others), you must try doing it high.

HEY HEY WE'RE THE MUNCHIES

It's a fact of high life: sometime after ingesting weed, users will be overwhelmed by the desire to eat everything. Known colloquially as "the munchies," "puff-n-stuff," and "involuntary mouthslaughter," the hunger that follows a high is brought on by THC's mimicking of the "hunger hormone" ghrelin, which instructs the body to seek out sustenance while increasing our ability to smell food (and driving us to eat more of it). Add to this weed's amplification of the sensual pleasures of taste and smell and you've got a perfect storm of biological drives conspiring to turn every stoner into an amateur competitive eater. Successful navigation of the munchies involves taking advantage of weed's luxurious food-enhancement properties without falling prey to the temptation to eat sixteen servings of everything. For more on munchie control, see Chapter 6: Maximizing Your Experience.

Unlike other psychoactive drugs, cannabis can't be categorized as simply a stimulant (like cocaine), a depressant (like alcohol), or a hallucinogen (like LSD). Instead, the effects of weed combine elements of all three categories.

On the "depressant" front, weed brings a reduction in stress and anxiety, ushering users into states of relaxation and diminished pain (thanks to cannabinoids' reduction of the number of pain messages sent to the body from the brain). Also affected: issues of physical coordination and perceptions of time and space. Avoid driving, performing surgery, and overconfidently descending staircases while high.

On the "stimulant" front, cannabis can flood users with feelings of energized well-being that border on euphoria. (It's not unusual for the face of a freshly high person to bear an inexplicable mile-wide smile.) With these feelings of well-being—brought about by cannabinoids' upping of dopamine and norepinephrine levels—comes a general heightening of sensory perception: colors are brighter, flavors are richer, jokes are funnier, cats are fluffier. For many users, weed produces a rush of creativity, rich with new ideas, speedy associations, and cohesive abstract thinking.

Beyond the simple depressant/stimulant divide lie marijuana's hallucinogenic properties, which are generally mild and make themselves known through an expansion of perception that seems to pull users into the eternal present, where they experience the world with fresh wonder and awe. However, in high doses—especially high doses of edibles, the THC of which is processed through the liver and turned into

superpowered 11-hydroxy-THC—weed can inspire something close to a baby LSD trip, complete with audiovisual hallucinations and epiphany-driven paralysis.

MEET *THE*
ENDOCANNABINOID SYSTEM!

For years, humanity enjoyed the effects of cannabis without
really understanding what weed did or how it did it. But in the
late 1980s, American researcher Allyn Howlett (along with
her graduate student–assistant William Devane) identified
receptors in the brain triggered specifically by cannabinoids,
suggesting the chemical compounds in weed mimic a naturally occurring brain chemical. (We wouldn't have receptors
waiting to be triggered by some outside weedy force, so weed
had to be mimicking an existing natural chemical.) Thus
brought the discovery of **endocannabinoids**—cannabinoids
produced naturally by our bodies—and the **endocannabinoid system**, a series of receptors throughout our brains and
bodies that exist to receive cannibinoids, be they endogenous
or delivered by bong.

Perhaps you're thinking: "Are you seriously saying God
or evolution or whatever rigged humanity with an internal
system for getting high?" The answer is yes, with scientists

positing the endocannabinoid system as an evolutionary development to help us cope—decreasing anxiety, improving mood, and modulating pain. (Less-than-fun fact: Science

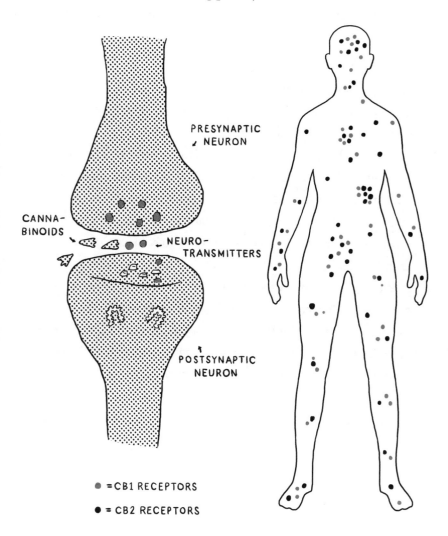

PRESYNAPTIC NEURON

CANNA-BINOIDS

NEURO-TRANSMITTERS

POSTSYNAPTIC NEURON

● = CB1 RECEPTORS

● = CB2 RECEPTORS

might have learned of the endocannabinoid system sooner if government-funded research allowed for investigation of weed's benefits, rather than focusing solely on why cannabis is a danger worthy of Schedule 1 classification alongside heroin.)

✑ WHEN CANNABINOIDS ATTACK ✑

Weed's pleasurable effects are brought on by cannabinoids' disruption of the brain's neural messaging—but "disrupting neural messaging" is an imprecise art, and different strains in different brains can create effects that cross the line from pleasant and fascinating to itchy and weird. For example, the neuron disruption that some users experience as expanded consciousness can trap others in a cul-de-sac of hypercritical introspection, and one person's THC-driven explosion of creative ideas can be another person's panic attack. The truth is that a good number of people who try weed experience predominately unpleasant effects, from intense anxiety to racing heart rates to crippling self-consciousness, and if you are one of these people, it is your right to never try weed again, no matter how persuasively it's pitched to you. Think of it like coffee: Some love it and can't imagine life without it, while others drink it and become insomniacs with diarrhea. (For more information, see Chapter 7: If You're High and Don't Like It.)

ON PARANOIA, OR WHY WON'T THAT DOG STOP JUDGING ME?

For a fair number of users, weed is a one-way ticket to paranoia, with roughly a quarter of recreational users experiencing anxiety, self-consciousness, judgmental introspection, and even panic attacks after ingesting THC. The reason for this highly predictable occurrence: dopamine, another naturally occurring chemical mimicked by THC, which can trick the brain into sending out errant warnings about threats of danger, making subjects unnerved by even the most common situations, from answering the phone to making eye contact with a dog. Why are some weed users transported to a land of peace and tranquility while others are cast into black holes of introspection? Blame the "entourage effect," wherein cannabinoids and terpenes bounce around individual brains to produce highly personal results. If you are someone who smokes weed and feels insane, admit you're cursed with a weed-hating brain and move on.

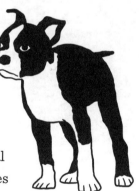

HE KNOWS WHAT YOU'RE THINKING, AND DOESN'T APPROVE.

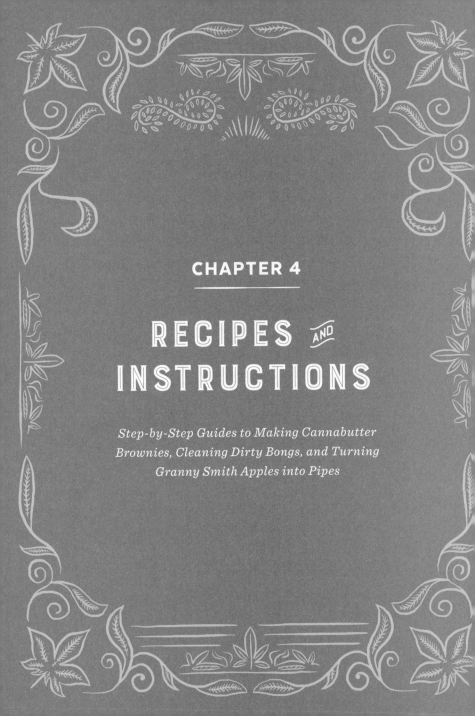

CHAPTER 4

RECIPES *and* INSTRUCTIONS

Step-by-Step Guides to Making Cannabutter
Brownies, Cleaning Dirty Bongs, and Turning
Granny Smith Apples into Pipes

I n this chapter you'll find step-by-step guides to executing an array of weed-based tasks, from cleaning dirty bongs to turning an apple into a pipe. But the majority of these tasks involve the kitchen—cooking cannabutter, baking weed brownies, making THC-infused cooking oil. Before we plunge into specifics of homemade marijuana edibles, allow me to shove the most important information right in your face.

DETERMINING THC DOSES IN HOMEMADE EDIBLES

Getting too high on homemade edibles is terrible and unfortunately super easy to do. Follow these tips to find a happy and manageable THC dose for your edibles.

1. **DETERMINE THE STRENGTH** of the weed you'll be cooking with. In Colorado, Washington, Oregon, and Alaska this means asking your salesperson, "What is the THC percentage of this weed?" People in prohibition states should operate on the assumption that most marijuana strains contain about 10 percent THC, which means a gram of cannabis contains roughly 100 milligrams of THC. (If you're dealing with high-octane hydroponic weed, the average should be 15 percent THC.)

2. **DO THE MATH.** The THC-dosing equation we'll be using comes from professional cannabis culinarian Jessica Catalano, who laid out the basics in her book *The Ganja Kitchen Revolution: The Bible of Cannabis Cuisine*. First, convert your amount of marijuana into milligrams of THC. (The cannabutter recipe calls for an eighth of an ounce of marijuana—that's 3.5 grams—which, at 100 milligrams THC per gram, means 350 milligrams of THC.) Then divide the THC-milligram number by the number of servings in the recipe (the "recipe yield"). The result is your per-serving THC dose.

CONVERTING MARIJUANA INTO MILLIGRAMS OF THC

For normal weed, assume 100 mg of THC per gram.
For high-grade weed, assume 150 mg per gram.

Eighth ounce = 3.5 grams
Quarter ounce = 7 grams
Half ounce = 14 grams
Ounce = 28 grams

3. For example, the brownie recipe calls for a stick of butter. One stick of our cannabutter contains 3.5 grams of weed/ 350 milligrams of THC. Typical THC doses are 5 to 10 milligrams for beginners, 20 to 30 milligrams for experienced users, and 40 to 60 milligrams for heavy users. With brownies cut into their recipe's yield of sixteen servings, each would contain 22 milligrams of THC—which is two and a half doses for a novice, a good dose for an intermediate, and half a dose for a heavy user.

DETERMINING THC DOSES IN HOMEMADE EDIBLES

EXPERIENCE LEVEL	DOSE
Beginner user	5 to 10 mg
Experienced user	20 to 30 mg
Heavy user	40 to 60 mg

4. Looking to further lower THC levels in your edibles? Try these tricks.

⭐ **UP YOUR RECIPE YIELD.** Back to our brownies: Instead of the recommended sixteen servings, cut the pan into twenty-four servings, each one of which will have a more navigable dose of 15 milligrams of THC. Or use a recipe with a naturally high yield—classic cookie recipes turn a stick of cannabutter into sixty cookies, each of which would have a reasonable 6 milligrams of THC per cookie.

⭐ **AIM FOR RECIPES THAT CALL FOR LESS BUTTER.** Instead of butter-dense brownies, consider making Rice Krispies Treats, which require a quarter of the butter used in brownies.

🌿 **CUT YOUR CANNABUTTER.** Just because a recipe calls for butter doesn't mean you have to use 100 percent cannabutter. Consider using half cannabutter and half regular butter.

EDIBLES RECIPES

CANNABUTTER

Cannabutter is butter infused with THC, the fat-soluble cannabinoid that's made psychoactive through its tussle with hot, fatty butter. Cannabutter is relatively easy to make and extremely easy to use; any recipe that calls for butter— brownies, cookies, pancakes, grilled cheese sandwiches, Alfredo sauce—can be made with cannabutter.

MAKES ABOUT ½ CUP CANNABUTTER

⅛ ounce (3.5 grams) cannabis

1 cup water, plus more as needed

½ cup (1 stick) unsalted butter

SPECIAL EQUIPMENT:

Electric grinder

15-by-15-inch cheesecloth

Rubber gloves

1. To prepare the cannabis, first remove any seeds and stems. Using an electric grinder, grind the cannabis into as fine a dust as possible.

2. In a medium saucepan, bring the water to a boil. Add the butter to the boiling water, then reduce the heat to low. Once the butter-water mixture is simmering—that means tiny rising bubbles and no more—add the ground cannabis, sprinkling it in slowly and stirring the mixture with a wooden spoon. Let the mixture simmer for 1 hour, stirring occasionally. Make sure the simmer never becomes a boil, and add extra water as needed to combat boil condensation. If your simmering mix ever looks more buttery than watery, add water. You don't want the butter to burn, which, like allowing a simmer to reach full boil, can damage precious cannabinoids.*

(continued)

---

* According to stoner lore, the longer you allow cannabutter to simmer, the richer it becomes in terpenes and so the greater its potency, with some users letting cannabutter simmer for up to twenty-four hours. However, the vast majority of cannabinoids are extracted within the first hour, and many users (this writer included) stick to a one-hour simmer. If you want to try an extended simmer, make it easy on yourself with a slow cooker.

3. Lay the cheesecloth across the bottom of a large heatproof glass bowl, letting the excess cloth hang over the sides. Carefully pour the butter-weed mixture into the cloth-lined bowl.

4. When the mixture is cool enough to be safely touched by rubber-gloved hands, put on rubber gloves, gather up the dry ends of cheesecloth, and begin squeezing the wad of hot, slimy plant material collecting at the bottom of your cheesecloth-straining contraption. Squeeze hard—you're aiming to force out every last bit of liquid, leaving a wad of dry-as-possible plant material in the cloth. When you're done, throw the leftover cannabis material in the garbage. It cannot help you now.

5. Allow the butter-weed mixture to cool on the counter for 1 hour or so, then cover the bowl with clear plastic wrap and place it in the refrigerator for at least 2 hours or let it set overnight.

6. As it cools, the THC-enhanced butter will harden into a waxy layer hovering above the funky leftover water.

When the butter has hardened in this way, remove the bowl from the fridge. Run a butter knife around the inside edge of the bowl to release the butter layer, which should now be pale green. Take a fork or slotted spoon and lift the butter layer from the bowl, placing it in a separate glass or plastic bowl. If it breaks into smaller pieces, that's fine— get all the buttery bits out of the bowl, then dispose of whatever gunky liquid is left. (And if it seems like there are tiny butter bits lurking in that leftover water, run it through a strainer on its way down the drain.)

7. Store the cannabutter in the fridge until you are ready to use it. (Cannabutter can be stored in a refrigerator for up to 2 months and retain its potency.)

PRO TIP: Direct high heat can damage cannabinoids, so use your cannabutter for baking rather than frying.

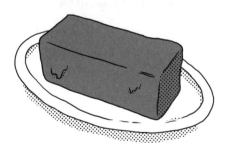

A-PLUS CANNABUTTER BROWNIES

So you've got cannabutter in hand and are ready to put it to use in some good old-fashioned pot brownies. Your primary step: finding a brownie recipe—or brownie box mix—that calls for *butter*. If you have a favorite vegetable oil–based brownie recipe that you want to spice up with weed, see Cannabis-Infused Cooking Oil on page 75.

If you're looking for a good butter-based box mix and live within twenty miles of a Trader Joe's, head directly there for a box of their inexpensive and delicious truffle brownie mix.

If you're looking to start from scratch and make the world's most delicious brownies that just happen to get you high, follow the recipe below, passionately recommended by my professional-baker sister-in-law, Mary, and adapted from Alice Medrich's Best Cocoa Brownies recipe from her book *Bittersweet*.

MAKES 16 (2-BY-2-INCH) BROWNIES

½ cup cannabutter
  (page 68)

2 tablespoons unsalted
  butter

¾ cup granulated sugar

½ cup brown sugar

¾ cup plus 2 tablespoons
  unsweetened cocoa
  powder

¼ teaspoon salt

½ teaspoon pure vanilla
  extract

2 large eggs, cold

½ cup all-purpose flour

¼ teaspoon baking powder

1. Preheat the oven to 325 degrees F, positioning the oven rack in the lower third of the oven.

2. Line the bottom and sides of an 8-by-8-inch baking pan with aluminum foil.

3. In a medium heatproof bowl, combine the butters, sugars, cocoa powder, and salt.

4. Fill a medium saucepan halfway with water and bring the water to a low simmer over low heat. (Simmer means a few tiny rising bubbles, and the heat should be as low as possible without ceasing to be a simmer.) Place the bowl of already-mixed ingredients inside the pan of barely simmering water, stirring occasionally, until the butter is melted and the mixture is smooth-ish and hot, 5 to 7 minutes. Remove the bowl from the pan and let it cool for a few minutes. (Note: For the next step, you want the mix warm, not hot, and if it looks suspiciously gritty, don't fret, it'll smooth out in the next step.)

5. Using a wooden spoon, stir in the vanilla. Add the eggs, one at a time, stirring vigorously after each addition, until the batter is thick, shiny, and smooth. Add the flour and baking powder, and stir until just combined, then vigorously beat the whole concoction for 1 more minute with a wooden spoon or rubber spatula.

(continued)

6. Spread the batter evenly in the prepared pan, and put the pan in the oven.

7. Bake for 20 to 25 minutes. When you can plunge a toothpick into the center of the tray and have it come out only lightly moist with batter, your brownies are ready to be removed from the oven.

8. Once cooled, cut the brownies into sixteen (2-by-2-inch) squares, and enjoy! If you made your cannabutter with run-of-the-mill weed, each brownie will have about 22 milligrams of THC. If you used THC-enhanced hydroponic, each brownie will have about 33 milligrams of THC. In either case, beginners will want to start with half a brownie.

WARNING: These brownies are freaking delicious, with flaky tops and moist centers, and you might be tempted to eat more than what constitutes your desired dosage. **PLEASE DON'T.** These brownies are drugs and must be treated as such. (For more information, see Determining THC Doses in Homemade Edibles on page 65.) If you want some of these freakily delicious brownies to enjoy during your "munchies" phase, make a supplementary batch with non-drugged butter, and label both drugged and non-drugged batches carefully.

CANNABIS-INFUSED COOKING OIL

Any oil you can think of—olive, canola, coconut, peanut, corn, baby—can be easily infused with THC, in a manner similar to Cannabutter (see recipe on page 68). With cannabis-infused cooking oil, the question is not so much "how?" but "why?" because cannabis oil can be a bit of a pain. First, there's the heat restriction—cannabis oil loses potency when subjected to above-medium heat, so using your THC oil to cook eggs over medium heat is fine, but wok-frying is not. Then there's the issue of dosing: It's not like you can have friends over for dinner, serve THC-spiked pesto salad, and expect everyone to have a harmonious THC-laced evening. Some guests might eat no pesto salad, others might eat seven servings, and whatever happens, users aren't going to feel effects until two hours later and for six hours after that.

Still, cannabis-enhanced oil can be perfect for many people, from medical marijuana patients who need regular dosing to stealth stoners attending family gatherings. (Keeping cookies away from others is way harder than warning people away from your "special gluten-free salad dressing.") Or maybe you just have a beloved brownie recipe that calls for oil instead of butter. Whatever the case, if you want to make cannabis-infused cooking oil, here's how.

MAKES ABOUT 1 CUP OIL

1 cup oil (olive, canola, coconut—whatever you want)	*SPECIAL EQUIPMENT:*
	Electric grinder
⅛ ounce (3.5 grams) cannabis	15-by-15-inch cheesecloth
	Rubber gloves

1. To prepare the cannabis, first remove any seeds and stems. Using an electric grinder, grind the cannabis into as fine a dust as possible.

2. In a medium saucepan or slow cooker on low heat, add the oil and heat it for 2 minutes. Sprinkle the cannabis into the oil, stirring throughout to make sure every fleck of weed is coated in the oil. Simmer on low heat, uncovered, for 45 minutes (or, if you're using a slow cooker, 2 hours), stirring occasionally.

CANNABIS OIL DOSAGE FACTS: This recipe involves an eighth of an ounce of weed—3.5 grams—being injected into one cup of oil. Each gram of weed has roughly 100 milligrams of THC, which means the full batch of oil contains 350 milligrams of THC, and each tablespoon of oil contains 33 milligrams of THC—a good dose for regular users, though newbies will want to start with a quarter of that.

3. While the oil simmers, lay the cheesecloth across the bottom of a large heatproof glass bowl, letting the excess cloth hang over the sides.

4. After simmering, remove the saucepan from the heat and carefully pour the oil mixture into the cloth-lined bowl.

5. When the mixture is cool enough to be safely touched by rubber-gloved hands, put on rubber gloves, gather up the dry ends of the cheesecloth, and begin squeezing the wad of hot, slimy plant material collecting at the bottom of your cheesecloth-straining contraption. Squeeze hard— you're aiming to force out every last bit of liquid, leaving a wad of dry-as-possible plant material in the cloth. When you're done, throw the leftover cannabis material in the garbage.

(continued)

6. Pour what's collected in the bowl into an opaque, airtight container—tinted glass bottles are best, but old plastic margarine tubs work well too—and refrigerate. The oil keeps its full potency for up to 2 months.

GRINDING 101

Throughout these recipes and instructions, users are instructed to grind weed. But not all grinds are the same, with certain tasks calling for certain grinds.

For joints and blunts, you'll want a coarse grind, with weed turned into nice soft flecks. (Inexpensive hand-held grinders do this type of grind perfectly.) You can also use an electric grinder if you're careful, making sure to stop after two or three quick bursts of grinding to ensure coarseness. If no grinder is available, there's the old penny trick (put weed nuggets in an empty pill bottle with a penny and shake) or just busting weed down by hand, breaking apart each bud with your fingers.

For cannabutter, tincture, and any other technique that involves submerging weed in liquid, you'll want the finest grind possible, which means using an electric grinder, such as a coffee grinder, blender, or food processor. (If you have trouble cleaning your grinder of sticky weed residue, give it a wipe with nontoxic Simple Green cleaner.)

Whatever your grinding technique, your bonus reward will be kief—the sticky THC-packed dust that gathers in a grinder through repeated use. The best grinders have a special bottom compartment specifically to gather kief, which can then be sprinkled in a joint or on a bowl and get you extra-special high.

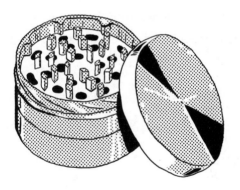

IF YOU REGULARLY ROLL JOINTS,
YOU'LL WANT A GRINDER.

CANNABIS TINCTURE

For people who enjoy getting high and don't mind the occasional terrible taste in their mouths, weed tinctures can be a wonderful thing. Essentially alcohol infused with THC, tinctures can be administered in two ways. The **sublingual method** involves squirting tincture under your tongue, where it tastes disgusting and rushes into your bloodstream, resulting in a high that lands almost as quickly as with smoking. The **masquerade method** involves squirting a dropperful of tincture into a strong-flavored liquid—orange juice, chocolate milk, V8—where the tincture's inherent grossness is subsumed in the dominant flavor, and the high lands one or two hours later.

MAKES ABOUT 1 CUP TINCTURE

¼ ounce (7 grams) of cannabis

1 cup high-proof alcohol (at least 90 proof—Everclear is best; cheap vodka will do)

SPECIAL EQUIPMENT:

Electric grinder

A quart canning jar with airtight lid

15-by-15-inch cheesecloth

Rubber gloves

Tinted glass tincture bottles with squeeze droppers (Find them at your health food store.)

PRO TIP: If your weed is moist, it'll be hard to grind, so dry it a bit by either leaving it out overnight or placing it between two pieces of toilet paper and giving it a blast with a hair dryer. (Do not microwave weed—it effs up the THC.)

1. Preheat oven to 240 degrees F.

2. To prepare the cannabis, first remove any seeds and stems. Using an electric grinder, grind the cannabis into as fine a dust as possible.

3. Spread the cannabis onto a 9-by-13-inch baking sheet and bake for 20 minutes. (This activates the THC in the cannabis you'll be turning into tincture by decarboxylating it.) Remove the baking sheet from the oven and let the cannabis cool for 30 minutes.

4. Place the cannabis into the canning jar, then add the alcohol. Screw the lid on tightly and give the jar some gentle shakes. Place the lidded jar in a cool, dark place. If there's room in the freezer, place it there. Most of the THC will be drawn into the liquid within a few hours, but you should let it stew for at least 24 hours for the full effects.

5. Lay the cheesecloth across the bottom of a large glass mixing bowl, letting the excess cloth hang over the sides. Give your jar a final shake, then carefully pour and strain

(continued)

the contents through the cheesecloth-prepared bowl. Put on rubber gloves and wring out as much liquid as you can—you're aiming to force out every last bit of liquid, leaving a wad of dry-as-possible plant material in the cloth. When you're done, throw the leftover cannabis material in the garbage.

6. Pour the liquid that's collected in your bowl into squeeze-dropper-topped bottles. (It's important to use opaque tinted bottles as they keep out THC-destroying light, and the dropper tops are key to dosing.)

CANNABIS TINCTURE DOSING FACTS: For best results, dose yourself from a one-ounce bottle. Following this recipe, each dropperful of a one-ounce bottle contains six milligrams of THC, making one dropper a nice dose for a beginner, three droppers good for an occasional user, and six droppers recommended for heavy users.

SMOKING INSTRUCTIONS

HOW TO ROLL A JOINT BY HAND

The ability to hand roll joints is a hard-earned skill with a degree of difficulty somewhere between driving a stick shift and playing castanets. Below are step-by-step instructions, rendered in sentences as clear as I can make them, alongside helpful illustrations. (If you need further guidance, consult a hand-rolled cigarette-smoking friend, or see Wiz Khalifa's video "How to Roll a Perfect Joint" at WizKhalifa.com.)

MAKES 1 JOINT

1 gram cannabis (see the gram-size outline on the following page)

1 rolling paper*

Manual handheld grinder (manual is best, but doing a quick, coarse grind with an electric grinder works too)

Semi-dexterous fingers

Saliva

(continued)

---

* The two main types are made of hemp and rice. Hemp papers are thicker, easier to grasp, and good for beginners. Rice papers are thinner, finer, and preferred by connoisseurs. (Standard-size papers are fine, but larger sizes can be more forgiving of beginner's klutziness.)

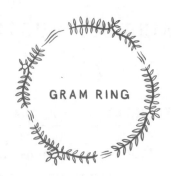

GRAM RING

1. To prep the cannabis, remove any seeds and stems, then give the weed a coarse grind. (Aim for nice soft flecks, rather than finely ground dust.)

2. Take the rolling paper and fold it in half lengthwise to create a weed-cradling crease. Keep the paper "sticky-side up," with the adhesive edge farthest away from you.

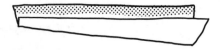

PRO TIP: Did you wind up with a joint that has an accidental tear, hole, or other flaw? Take a spare rolling paper, rip off its gummed glue strip, and use it as a bandage!

3. Spread the weed along the crease in the paper. Poke the weed flakes around with your fingertips to achieve equal distribution along the paper.

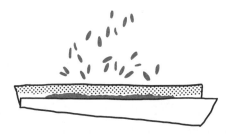

4. With the thumb and index finger of your right hand, pick up the joint by pinching its upper edges. (Imagine a stork carrying a bundled baby.) Place your joint baby in your left hand, holding it in a pinchy makeshift cradle formed by your thumb and first two fingers. Form an identical thumb-and-first-two-fingers cradle with your right hand, with one end of the fledgling joint in each hand.

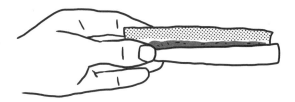

(continued)

5. Rolling your joint does not mean rolling it up—not yet. For now, the rolling maneuver is a gentle rolling back and forth, a movement that softens up your paper while perfecting the distribution of your weed and condensing it into a joint-like mass.

6. Once you've achieved your desired joint shape through back-and-forth rolling, it's wrapping time. Tuck the nonadhesive edge of the paper down into the joint, then press lightly with your thumbs and use your index fingers to roll the joint up tight, leaving only the gummy glue strip exposed.

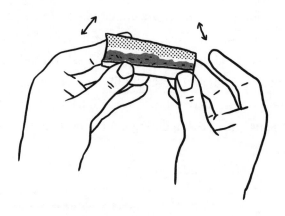

7. Run your tongue along the gummy glue strip and commence your final roll, ending by pressing your saliva-moistened glue strip down to seal your now-finished joint.

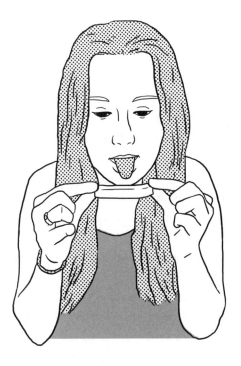

PRO TIP: Is your joint lightly wet from an overzealous glue lick? Run a lighter's flame up and down the length of your joint, quickly enough that nothing catches fire but everything dries out and tightens up.

SPRUCE UP JOINTS
WITH A ROACH TIP!

If smoking joints is a regular thing for you, you'll want to familiarize yourself with the roach tip, which is a small strip of paper that's been folded and rolled into filter-like shape that's inserted at the inhalation end of a joint, where it helps keep air flowing freely, prevents flecks of weed from entering users' mouths, and allows a joint to be smoked down to its weedy end without singeing anyone's lips.

To make a roach tip, you'll need a strip of plain, non-glossy paper approximately a half-inch wide by three inches long. (A strip cut from an index card works perfectly.) At one end of your strip, make the smallest fold you can manage—an eighth of an inch or so—then fold this eighth-inch fold in on itself three times. Once you've got your four tight folds, roll up the rest of the paper tightly around this foundation, and insert your finished roach tip at one end of your rolling paper, rolling it up along with your weed to make your built-in roach-tipped joint.

PRO TIP: Do not make a roach tip out of glossy magazine paper (you'll regret the smell of it burning) or repurpose a filter from a cigarette, which absorbs too much of weed's fun stuff.

STEP 1

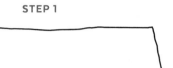

STEP 2

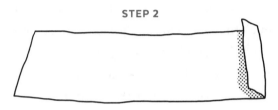

STEP 3

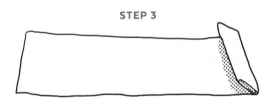

STEP 4

HOW TO ROLL A JOINT
WITH A ROLLING MACHINE

If you want to smoke a joint without mastering the intricate skill of hand-rolling, get yourself an inexpensive cigarette-rolling machine and live happily ever after. Available at most convenience stores and all smoke shops, rolling machines involve the placement of both weed and paper in a U-shaped bin, on which the roller bars apply such uniform pressure the resulting joint is virtually indistinguishable from a commercially manufactured cigarette. (This can be helpful camouflage, if you live in a state where that matters.)

MAKES 1 JOINT

A cigarette-rolling machine

1 rolling paper (whether they're hemp or rice doesn't matter, but get the standard size to fit the rolling machine)

1 gram cannabis

Semi-dexterous fingers

Saliva

1. Prep the rolling machine. A rolling machine has two positions: open (with roller bars spread wide) and closed (with rollers placed side by side). To begin, set your machine to the open position.

2. To prep the cannabis, remove any seeds and stems, then give the weed a coarse grind. (Aim for nice soft flecks, rather than finely ground dust.)

3. Spread the cannabis along the rolling machine's vinyl cradle, aiming for equal distribution of weed along the length of the cradle.

4. Close the roller by moving the lower bar to the closed position, enclosing your weed in the cradle. Once closed, give the rollers a couple spins with your thumbs and forefingers, rolling toward yourself. (This will solidify your weed into a helpful joint-like mass.)

5. Keeping the rolling machine closed, insert the non-gummed edge of the rolling paper into the slit between the rollers. Make sure the gummed edge is facing up, toward you. Using your thumbs and forefingers, roll the paper down into the machine, rolling toward yourself and stopping when only the gummed edge of the paper is left exposed.

(continued)

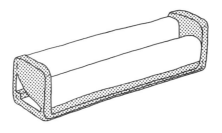

6. Lick the gummy adhesive edge of the paper, and using your thumbs and forefingers, give the joint a final couple of rolls, rolling toward yourself and applying light pressure. (Your goal is to make sure the adhesive strip gets tamped into place.) Warning: It is entirely possible to roll a joint so tightly that it's unsmokable. Use a light touch so air can flow.

7. Open the rolling machine and meet your new joint.

HOW TO ROLL A BLUNT

Blunts are joints rolled in cigar papers, which are made of tobacco and thus contain nicotine. Cigar papers are available in packs at smoke shops, but many users simply repurpose the paper of a commercially produced, purchased-at-a-convenience-store cigar. (Optimos are popular.)

MAKES 1 BLUNT

1 to 2 grams of cannabis (a blunt uses roughly double the weed of a joint)	Manual handheld grinder
	Knife or razor blade
Cigar papers or a store-bought cigar	Saliva
	Lighter

1. To prep the weed, remove any seeds and stems, then give the cannabis a coarse grind.

2. Prep the paper. If using readymade cigar rolling papers, crease the paper lengthwise down the middle with the gummy-side up. If repurposing a store-bought cigar, take your blade and cut the cigar lengthwise down its side. Carefully pry the cigar open and scoop out the insides. (Be careful—dried tobacco leaves are unsurprisingly fragile.)

3. Spread your weed evenly down the length of your cigar papers and follow steps 4 to 7 in How to Roll a Joint by Hand (pages 85 to 86) to finish your blunt.

4. With a repurposed cigar, you don't have the luxury of a gummy adhesive strip to make your blunt stay shut. Instead, you'll just have to give your repurposed-cigar blunt a good spitty lick at the sealing point, then "bake" it closed by running a lighter's flame up and down the length of the blunt.

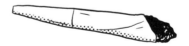

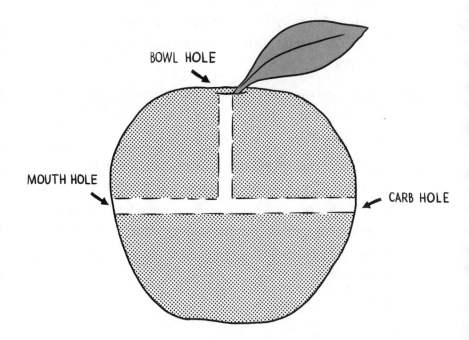

BOWL HOLE

MOUTH HOLE

CARB HOLE

HOW TO TURN AN APPLE INTO A PIPE

Because sometimes you find yourself with weed with no other way to smoke it.

Fresh, crisp apple
(freshness is key—a soft
apple might collapse
during stabbing)

Ballpoint pen you don't
mind ruining (classic Bic
style with removable ink
tube is best)

Some weed

Aluminum foil (optional)

1. Remove the apple's stem. Make sure you get the entire stem. Dig if you have to. (If the root of the stem is being stubborn, go after it with a key.)

2. Remove the cap and ink column from the ballpoint pen.

3. Jam the pen casing down into the apple through the stem hole, stopping when you're midway through and have created a tunnel roughly ¼-inch wide from the top of the apple to its center. Discard any apple-jamming refuse that may be stuck in the pen.

4. On the side of your apple, as close to the center as possible, stab a hole that goes all the way through the apple—running straight through the center like an arrow and

(continued)

connecting to the bottom of your first tunnel. (If making this connection requires supplemental tunneling, do it.) Your apple will now have two holes at its sides and one on top. One of the side holes is the mouthpiece. The other is the carb. The hole on top is your bowl.

5. Add the weed and smoke. If your weed is in sturdy bud form, rest it on the hole on top of the apple, put your mouth over one side hole and a finger over the other, hit your weed with fire, and inhale. (After a few seconds, uncover the carb hole.) If your weed is loose and shaky, make an impromptu screen with aluminum foil, placing the foil over the apple's top hole, then poking it with a toothpick or safety pin to create a half-dozen suction holes.

6. Contrary to what your cousin told you, eating a pipe apple after use will not get you high. It will only make you awesome.

HOW TO USE A BONG

1. Let's start by identifying a bong's parts. As you can see in the illustration on the following page, the bowl is where the weed goes, the mouthpiece is what you inhale from, and the chamber is what fills with smoke as you inhale. The stem holds the bowl, and somewhere on a bong there's a carburetion point—typically, it's either a small "carb hole" placed midway down the back of the chamber (allowing easy coverage with a thumb), or it's a "pull carb," wherein air is let into the chamber by lifting the bowl out of the stem. (Pull carbs are usually found on glass bongs, and carb holes are usually found on plastic bongs.)

2. Fill your clean bong with ¼ cup or so fresh tap water, pouring the water down through the mouthpiece into the chamber. (If the bong's got a carb hole, cover it while pouring.) You'll want a couple of water resting at the bottom of the bong's chamber. Make sure there's enough for the lower end of the stem to be fully submerged in water. (If your bong is not yet clean, skip to How to Clean a Bong on page 100 and come back.)

3. If your weed's in nice big bud form, grab a bud and shove it in the bowl. If you've got flaky shake, take a pinch and drop it in. (And if you're using superfine ground weed, make sure your bowl has a screen.)

(continued)

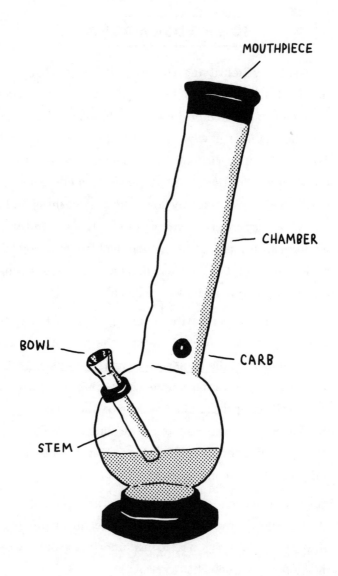

MOUTHPIECE

CHAMBER

BOWL

CARB

STEM

4. To take a hit, pick up the bong and, if it's got a carb hole, cover it with your thumb. Hold a flame to the weed in the bowl while inhaling through the mouthpiece and keeping your thumb over the carb hole. Inhaled smoke will rise in the chamber, and when you're ready for that smoke to rush into your lungs, remove your thumb from the carb hole (or if you're dealing with a pull carb, slide the bowl from the stem). Fresh air will rush into the chamber and send the smoke rushing into your face.

5. Cover your cough. The only shame in coughing is flying saliva. (If your cough continues, drink some water.)

6. Want a big hit? Don't release the carb until the chamber's dense with smoke. (Use as many inhalations as you need to get the smoke density you crave. Smoke will keep collecting in the chamber until the carb is released.) Want a small hit? Release the carb as soon as the first wisp of smoke rises in the chamber. Whatever size hit you take, it should end with you inhaling everything in the chamber, leaving the bong free of smoke for the next person. Change your bong's water on a daily basis. It gets gross fast.

CLEANING INSTRUCTIONS

HOW TO CLEAN A BONG

After a few uses, a bong will begin to collect a sticky brown residue along the inside of its chamber. This resinous residue is easy to clean away in its fledgling stages, but left untended it can grow into a thick black sludge that's such a disgusting chore to clean you'll consider throwing out your bong and starting over with a fresh one. This is dumb and expensive, so don't let your bong go too long without a cleaning. Once residue becomes visible, it's time for a quick cleaning.

Optional: rubber bands, plastic wrap, rubber gloves

1¾ cups isopropyl alcohol (a.k.a. rubbing alcohol), divided, plus more as needed

9 tablespoons kosher salt, divided, plus more as needed

Pipe cleaners

2 ziplock bags (sandwich-size)

1. Remove your bong's bowl and dump the old bong water down the toilet. (Never dump bong-related liquids down sinks. Resin is too nasty.)

2. Make the bong as watertight as possible. Some people make do with a thumb over the stem hole and a palm

over the mouthpiece (with or without rubber gloves), while others seal the stem and mouthpiece with plastic wrap held tight with rubber bands, placing supplementary wrap over the carb hole. Whatever the method, make sure you wind up with a bong that can be semi-filled with liquid, shaken briskly, and not leak salty alcohol sludge everywhere.

3. Add 3 tablespoons of the salt and ¼ cup of the isopropyl alcohol to your empty bong.

4. Shake your alcohol-and-salt-spiked bong for a full minute. Set a timer. You may get bored and even tired. Keep going. The alcohol helps dissolve the sticky resin, the salt acts as an abrasive, and you are the engine that makes the whole thing work.

5. After shaking, dump the sludgy alcohol-salt solution down the toilet and flush it away. If the bong still has patches of grime, repeat steps 3 to 6 as many times as necessary. (If you clean when residue is light, one pass will do the trick.)

(continued)

6. Rinse the chamber with hot water and enjoy your good-as-new bong.

7. Your bong's bowl and stem will also need to be cleaned. To do this, place the bowl in one ziplock bag and the stem in another. To each bag add 3 tablespoons of the salt and ¾ cup of the isopropyl alcohol. Let the pieces soak in the salty alcohol bags for 10 minutes, then get to shaking. Shake and repeat until pieces are clean. Dump crud water down the toilet.

8. Beyond full cleaning there's the smaller issue of a clearing a bowl that's become clogged with ash and resin and accumulated gunk. For this, you'll want a slender metal scraping device—head shops sell official scraping tools, but a paper clip bent to straight works fine.

PRO TIP: All resinous gunk is easier to deal with when its warmed up, so give your dirty bowl a blast with a lighter before getting down to poking and scraping.

HOW TO CLEAN A PIPE

Your pipe's material determines how it will be cleaned. To clean a wooden pipe, you'll need a lighter, pipe cleaners, and some sort of poking tool. (Smoke shops sell great little metal pokers, but a bent paper clip works okay too.) First, loosen the pipe's interior gunk by drawing a flame through it—hold a lighter over the (empty) bowl and suck through the mouthpiece. After you've done this a few times, start digging—first with your poking tool, then with a pipe cleaner. Dig out all the resin that's collected in your bowl. Run your poking tool along the sides of the bowl and stem to scrape off gathered goopy resin, depositing what you scrape free onto a paper towel. For a final step, run a pipe cleaner all the way through your pipe, then do it five more times.

Metal, glass, and ceramic pipes can be cleaned via the method first mentioned in How to Clean a Bong on page 100—place dirty pieces in ziplock sandwich-size bags full of rubbing alcohol and salt and shake until clean. Another method involves boiling the dirty pieces in water on the stove, which works great for metal pipes, can work fine for glass pipes (but be sure to place your pipe in the water *before* it boils and leave it there until the water cools to room temperature), and should be avoided with ceramic pipes. If you choose this method, pick up a cheap saucepan at Goodwill that you'll use for only purposes of pipe-boiling, and add ½ cup of salt to your boiling water before putting in your piece. After boiling, turn off the heat and let the piece sit in the water for two minutes, after which you should remove the piece with tongs and let it continue to cool on a paper towel on the counter. (Don't rinse just-boiled glass pieces in cool water, which could cause them to shatter.) Whichever method you use, finish up by doing detail work with your poking tool and pipe cleaners, and if your pipe uses a screen, put in a fresh one.

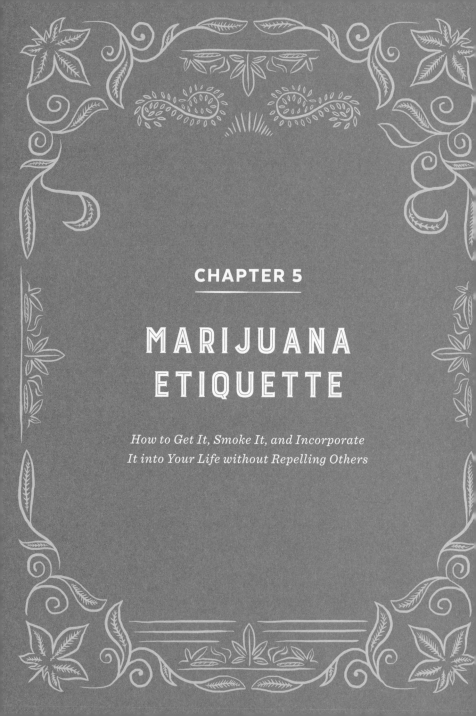

CHAPTER 5

MARIJUANA ETIQUETTE

*How to Get It, Smoke It, and Incorporate
It into Your Life without Repelling Others*

Like any recreational endeavor, smoking weed comes with its own set of customary rules for polite use. Many of these customs are perennials that apply across all areas of life: Cover your cough. Say please and thank you. Mind your stink. No means no. But a whole bunch of other weed customs involve intricate dances around issues of money, status, and legality, and this chapter will teach you the steps.

WEED: GETTING IT

Attaining marijuana is a task that's defined by where you live. For residents of Colorado, Washington, Alaska, Oregon, and whatever the next state to legalize the commercial sale of recreational marijuana may be, getting weed is as simple as going to the store. For all others, it's a tricky errand involving word-of-mouth contacts, light engagement with the underworld, and serious flexibility and deference.

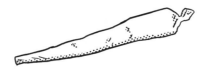

DEALING DEALERS

Dealers are wonderful humans who take the legal risk of buying weed in quantities large enough to sell smaller amounts to recreational users. Dealers can range from textable bike messengers who make house calls (viva NYC!) to purposeful park loiterers whispering "420" to passersby. Most often, a dealer is a casual acquaintance—a friend of a friend, or at least an acquaintance of an acquaintance—whose presence in your life is for the sole purpose of selling you weed.

This is less simple and more intimate than it sounds. At the center of the dealer-buyer relationship lies a basic imbalance of power: the dealer takes the greater legal risk and claims a quasi-monopoly on supply (if buyers had another good way to get weed, they wouldn't be looking for a dealer), while the buyer is left largely defenseless (disgruntled customers can't call the Better Business Bureau or police). But out of this uneven ground can grow perfectly cordial, mutually beneficial relationships, so long as potential buyers take care to protect themselves and respect their dealers.

⌐ FINDING A DEALER ⌐

For potential buyers looking for dealers, word-of-mouth is pretty much the best and only hope. And since most people don't run around blabbing about their weed purchases, asking the right questions at the right time is key. Say you've been invited to join in on some weed puffery at a party: Blurting out "Can you help me get some of my own?" is gauche. But accepting the invitation, enjoying the puff, and, if the time feels right, asking fellow participants if anyone knows a dealer looking for new customers, is perfectly acceptable and exactly how 99 percent of smokers found their weed sources. (Alternate methods: Take a loaf of banana bread to your neighbors with the occasional weed smell escaping from their apartment, and if they seem nice and helpful, ask if they know how you might acquire such a smell for your own place; or move to Colorado, Washington, Alaska, or Oregon, and go to the store.)

⸎ KEEPING A DEALER ⸎

So you've found a dealer you like who sells you weed you love—now it's your job to not fuck it up. Why is it *your* job? Because of that aforementioned imbalance of power, which allows dealers to be messy, tardy, and temperamental in ways that are off-limits to buyers, who must jump through dueling hoops of precision and flexibility. Not only must buyers be prepared to show up to dealer meetings on time with correct change, they must roll with the punches if the plan falls through, or if a dealer shows up four hours late and needs to use your bathroom, or insists on showing you forty-five minutes of *Hobbit* DVD outtakes before getting around to selling you anything.

Lucky for all, most weed dealers—most of the ones I've dealt with, at least—are sane, sensible humans, often with non-black-market jobs, who happen to sell weed on the side. As such, the onus placed on buyers typically involves less masochistic deference to unreliable dealer-tyrants and more behavioral precision. The basics:

🌿 **BE HONEST, PUNCTUAL, AND RELIABLE.** These traits combine to create trustworthiness, which is the key component of a good buyer-dealer relationship. In a black-market marijuana transaction, both buyer and seller are placed in a vulnerable position legally, and both sides prefer to take this risk with a responsible adult.

🌿 **BE FLEXIBLE.** Remember when I mentioned how dealers can sometimes be flaky and buyers just have to suck it up? It's true, and smart buyers can up their chances for happiness by avoiding tight situations. Plan ahead so you can leisurely contact your dealer about "a good time to meet up in the next couple days," rather than calling with an abrupt, desperate "Can I come over now?" Speaking of timing: you'll find a happier dealer as the one person reaching out on a weekday afternoon than you will as one of dozens frantically texting on Friday evening.

✷ **BE DISCREET.** Contrary to lore, weed dealers don't appreciate being hit with glaringly euphemistic questions about "fuzzy green sweaters," "420," or other dumb code that doesn't fool anyone. Dealers know why customers are calling, so communications can generally be restricted to issues of when and where to meet. "Up for a visit?" is a good pitch to a stay-at-home dealer, while one who makes house calls can be approached with "Hi! Hoping to find a time for you swing by." Extend your discretion through all phases of your weed purchase. (For example, if you're visiting your dealer, don't park in a loading zone with your hazard lights on or approach the building with cash in hand. Park like a normal person and keep your money in your pants till you are behind closed doors.)

✷ **BRING CORRECT CHANGE.** If you're looking to buy a small amount—say, five dollars' worth—make sure you've got a five-dollar bill or five ones. If you're wanting to spend fifty dollars, don't show up with three twenties from the ATM and expect change. Go to the convenience store, buy the Almond Snickers you'll be so happy to have later with a twenty-dollar bill, and get the exact change you need.

✷ **ONCE YOU'VE FOUND A DEALER WITH GOOD PRODUCT, CONSIDER BUYING LARGER AMOUNTS.** At the beginning of a new dealer-buyer relationship, a five- or ten-dollar purchase is understandable—you're figuring out what's what. But once you've determined your dealer has product you like, consider buying in larger amounts—say, fifty dollars and up. This benefits everyone: customers typically get a lower per-gram price the more grams they buy, and dealers don't get put through the whole text-call-meetup rigmarole to sell some piddly amount. (For more, see How Much Weed Should I Buy? on the opposite page.)

✳ **TIP YOUR DEALER FOR ABOVE-AND-BEYOND SERVICE.** Generally you can assume your dealer sets his or her prices in a way that ensures a reasonable profit, so tipping for a basic transaction isn't typical. But if your dealer jumps through hoops—say, meeting you on super-short notice in the lobby of the office where you work—a small tip is appropriate. (Nothing crazy—don't go tipping 20 percent on a three hundred dollar ounce of weed. Just toss 'em a few extra bucks to say thanks.)

HOW MUCH WEED
SHOULD I BUY?

The basic measurements you'll be dealing with are grams and ounces. One gram of quality weed will get you and a friend nicely high for an evening, and most folks don't bother their dealers unless they're looking to buy at least 3.5 grams, a.k.a. an eighth of an ounce (popularly abbreviated to "an eighth"). Larger serving sizes include the quarter ounce (7 grams), the half ounce (14 grams), and the ounce—28 full grams that is sometimes called a "zip," as one ounce of weed comfortably fills a standard ziplock sandwich bag, turning it into a puffy green pillow. For casual users, an eighth is a sensible purchase, giving you some for now, some for later, and some to stash away for rainy days and houseguests.

GOOD WEED
VS. BAD WEED

How can you tell if the weed you're about to buy is any good? Use your senses. If weed looks brown and brittle, is loaded with sticklike stems, and smells like nothing, it's crud.

All good weed is green, with just a few sticky stems (always attached to a bud) and a pungent smell. Some dealers will offer to let the customer have a sample puff on-site, which is very nice, but requires the sampler to either drive home high or stick around till the high wears off, which can result in mandatory viewings of Sasquatch documentaries and questionable make-out sessions.

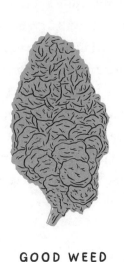

GOOD WEED

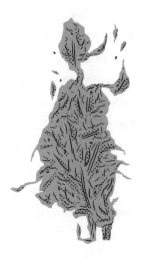

BAD WEED

SHOPPING FOR LEGAL WEED AND WEED-RELATED PARAPHERNALIA

If you are lucky, someday you will find yourself in a state that permits the legal sale of recreational marijuana. (For now, these states are Colorado, Washington, Alaska, and Oregon, but be patient.) While in these states, you will have the opportunity to patronize an actual store that sells marijuana—and you must seize it. For serious weed fans, the first visit to a legal marijuana dispensary—where acres of high-quality artisan weed glistens in glass gallon jars, alongside cigar-size joints and every marijuana-enhanced product you can imagine—can be like waking up in some magical Narnia-Disneyland-Heaven; there may be light, soft crying. (However, for those with loved ones serving mandatory prison sentences for selling negligible amounts of weed, there might be an urge to riot.) And for marijuana novices, there are 1,001 easy opportunities to blast your face off with mega-powerful weed, which is often counterintuitively and treacherously packaged in deeply familiar and benign forms, like a chocolate-chip cookie.

It is the moral duty of every marijuana novice and/or lightweight to identify themselves as such upon entering a legal marijuana dispensary, particularly in regard to marijuana edibles. Say it loudly and proudly: "I am a marijuana wuss and I do not want to get so high that I think I'm already dead so please give me serious guidance about strength and dosage." (See dosing information in Chapter 4: Recipe & Instructions.)

Speaking of shopping, no matter what state you reside in, you might have occasion to patronize a "smoke shop," "head shop," or "tobacco store" to purchase a tool for smoking marijuana—a bong or a pipe. Such stores have weird restrictions and superstitions, so when you are shopping for a marijuana bong, you should never speak the words *marijuana* or *bong*. If you are shopping for a pipe to smoke weed out of, you are shopping simply for "a pipe." If you a shopping for a bong, you are shopping for a "water pipe." I repeat, never mention marijuana in a store that sells tools that might be used for smoking marijuana.

WEED: SMOKING IT
a.k.a. the fun part

Etiquette regarding the smoking of marijuana is specific to the role you play in the smoking experience: host (the person in possession of weed who's inviting others to join in) or guest (the person being offered weed).

✿ HINTS FOR HOSTS! ✿

✤ **KEEP YOUR BONG, PIPE, AND ASHTRAYS AS NON-DISGUSTING AS POSSIBLE.** Due to the nature of burning material, bongs, pipes, and ashtrays are doomed to become gross and smelly. But they don't need to stay that way. Clean the gunk out of your pipe with a pipe cleaner. (Duh.) Scrape your bowls clean with a malfangled paper clip or official scraping tool acquired at a not-a-marijuana Smoke Shop. Dump out your ashtrays and scrub 'em like dirty plates. Subject your bong to the cleaning regimen detailed on page 100. Every one of these tasks will be mildly annoying to perform on a regular basis, but you must, for the rewards are plentiful. A sparkling clean bong can make any old stoner feel like a pampered duchess.

✤ **DE-SEED YOUR WEED.** This means removing any and all of the tiny pale-green seeds that occasionally dot a pot purchase. When left in weed and smoked, these seeds release a blandly nauseating taste into your otherwise delicious pipe or bong hit. Seeding your weed takes some precise attention—seeds are good hiders—but it's crucial. You don't need to dig through every new bag of weed searching for seeds—eight out of ten bags won't have 'em—but if you see one seed, you can expect to find more, so get to seeding.

✤ **DE-STEM YOUR WEED TOO.** Stems in weed range from the sticklike mini-branches that anchor big conglomerates of buds to the tiny stubs protruding from the top of individual nuggets, and wherever you find them, you should strip them away and throw them out. Even though they're green and can smell weedy, stems produce negligible psychoactive effects, taste disgusting, and often bestow wicked headaches.

✸ **GIVE THE FIRST HIT TO A GUEST.** After you pack your de-seeded and de-stemmed weed in your pipe or bong, offer the first hit to someone else. This is an old stoner tradition, and it's a nice one, so let's keep it going. (If you happen to be the guest recipient of the first hit, aim to make sure the second hitter is the host.)

✸ **GIVE A WARNING ABOUT YOUR WEED'S STRENGTH.** Weed can range from backyard ragweed to hyperdosed super-strains, so you should give smokers some idea of what they should expect. "Start with a small hit" is never bad advice.

✸ **STRIVE TO BE CONSIDERATE.** Timing is key for social smoking. Typically, not everybody at a gathering will be interested in partaking, and some may not enjoy being around a bunch of high people. Play it by ear. Sometimes stepping outside for a puff before sitting down at a dinner party is the most natural thing in the world; other times, it's completely inappropriate. The ideal is to have any and all weed usage fit into the proceedings in a manner similar to alcohol, not overwhelm everything with invasive smells and serious mood alterations. Even in your own home, aim to smoke either outdoors or in an enclosed, pot-specific space—you don't want your secondhand pot smoke to complicate the workplace drug tests of innocent bystanders.

THE "GREEN HIT"

The "green hit" is the first draw taken from a freshly packed bowl, where the flame makes the first burnt mark on a perfect field of green. If you are the recipient of the green hit, aim the flame at a corner of the bowl, rather than torching dead center—this will preserve a subsequent greenish hit for someone drawing on the opposite side of the bowl.

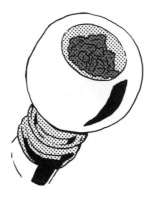

ॐ GUIDANCE FOR GUESTS! ॐ

So you've been invited to smoke someone else's weed. Lucky you! Here's how to proceed:

✴ **IF YOU FEEL LIKE BEING HIGH, SAY "YES, PLEASE"** and don't let anyone shame you about your decision. If you don't feel like being high, say "No, thank you" and don't let anyone shame you about your decision.

✴ **ASK ABOUT STRENGTH.** If your host doesn't naturally offer the information, ask him or her about the potency of the weed you're about to imbibe.

✴ **KEEP IT DRY.** Smoking weed involves putting your mouth on the mouthpiece of a pipe or bong, and—spoiler alert—human mouths contain saliva. Should you happen to get some of your saliva on the mouthpiece of a pipe or bong, give it a wipe with your sleeve or a napkin and send the pipe or bong on its way. Don't be shy about wiping. If you're too embarrassed to publicly acknowledge your own spit, you'll be fatally wounded by the shit people say behind your back after you pass them a spitty bong.

✴ **HIT IT AND QUIT IT.** Whether you're using a pipe, a bong, or a joint, guests should take a single hit—one midsize inhalation—and pass the device along. If your host is like 99.9 percent of marijuana hosts throughout history, that pipe/bong/joint will come around again, and again, and maybe again, and novice smokers should aim to recuse themselves from proceedings earlier than later—seasoned smokers can keep a bong going to a point that would paralyze a novice. (For more information, see the glossary entry for Bogarting on page 173.)

🌿 **CLEAR THE CHAMBER.** When smoking from a bong, after you take your midsize hit, make sure you've inhaled all the smoke from the chamber before passing the bong to the next person. You don't need to suck down the entire chamberful of smoke in one draw—typically, your initial draw will get 90 percent of the smoke into your lungs. Once this (and any attendant coughing) is done, inhale whatever stray smoke is left in the chamber and pass it along.

🌿 **CHIP IN.** People share their marijuana because it's a great pleasure to do so, and guests let hosts indulge in this great pleasure (while also getting high on someone else's weed). If you find yourself with a reliable marijuana benefactor, consider ways you might play a part in the experience—bring a supplementary stash of weed, show up with cheese and a baguette or a bottle of sparkling water, or just toss a five-dollar bill stuck with a sticky note that says "Thank you" on a countertop. Stoners share because they love to, but it's always nice to have generosity acknowledged, so refrain from visiting a stoner-host friend bearing anything less than a lightly refrigerated box of Junior Mints (and nothing more than a bottle of wine or six-pack of craft beer).

EDIBLES ETIQUETTE

If, in your role as host, you decide to make marijuana-laced edibles available to guests, it is your duty to either keep all edibles hidden and available on an offered-directly-by-you basis, or leave edibles out for public consumption and make sure they're so clearly marked—for example, "DANGER: DRUGGED BROWNIES!"—that not even the dunciest dunce could mistake them for regular food. And if you ever have an idea to "accidentally" serve THC-enhanced anything to anyone, punch yourself in the face until subdued. Anyone on the receiving end of such an accidental dosing has every right to unfriend you forever and perhaps press charges, so don't get cute.

AVOIDING DETECTION

At every stage of its being, from skunky nuggets in a baggie to acrid smoke in the air, weed stinks, and it's every weed smoker's duty to minimize the effect this stink has on innocent bystanders (including landlords and cops).

The battle against weed-stink starts as soon as you leave your dealer's place with a skunky bag of weed, which you should immediately place in an airtight container. The cheap plastic stuff you use for kitchen leftovers is perfect. (However, once you get your weed home, both the plastic baggie and plastic container should be ditched for something better. See What's the Best Way to Store Weed? on page 128.)

When it comes to smoking weed, the number-one best way to avoid the classic, room-dominating stink is to use a vaporizer, which emits only a whisper of scent that dissipates quickly and is not remotely weedy. But if you insist on actual weed smoking, with all its gross and glorious smoke and fire and stink, it's your job to keep your hot smoky mess reasonably contained. The fact is that some people hate the smell of pot smoke as much as other people hate the smell of cigars or cigarettes or indoor spray-paint or any other heavy intrusive stink, and the more you do to protect others from your weed stink, the better.

Live in a house by yourself or with fellow weed smokers? Feel free to smoke inside wherever you feel safe doing so. One of weed's many miraculous traits is that even its heaviest stink steadily dissipates. Unlike chemical-laden cigarette smoke, which clings to surfaces with a permanence that feels archival, even the heaviest weed smoke goes on its way in a day or two. Strive to be considerate—clouding up your enclosed living room is better than having a fan blow smoke out a window toward your neighbors.

Live in an apartment, condo, or similarly close-knit situation? The stink-containing demands placed on you are greater than those placed on single-occupancy house dwellers. Key to your mission is sparing your neighbors the annoyance of having to confront you about your stinky weed. No one likes bugging neighbors about stuff, and weed makes it extra weird. (Your neighbors may be full-time lobbyists for federal marijuana legalization, but that doesn't mean they want your weed stink wafting into their lives on a regular basis.)

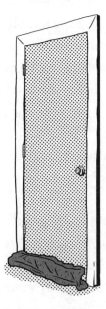

The basics for responsibly smoking in an enclosed space have remained the same since the first Cro-Magnon freshman flared up in his cave-dorm: Place a damp towel along the bottom of the door connecting your smoking area to the larger world. Smoke near an open window (but don't blow smoke directly out). For extra credit, take an empty toilet-paper or paper-towel roll, stuff it with dryer sheets, and exhale your weed smoke through that. (What comes out still smells lightly gross, but it's way less potty than regular pot smoke.)

SMOKE-PROOF A ROOM
WITH A DOOR-CRACK TOWEL!

Places of residence aren't the only vectors for weed stink worth worrying about. Sometimes the smoky stink of weed can envelop entire humans, and you should strive to avoid being one of them. Puffing in a car before heading into a restaurant/opera/baby shower? Leave time to take a stroll or two around the block to air out, while sucking on some Certs. Puffing a joint before a party? Make sure you've got an airtight container for your roach (a plastic sandwich-size ziplock bag is perfect) and hit the bathroom to wash your hands as soon as you arrive—joints can stink up fingers something fierce. Prone to bloodshot eyes post-smoking? Invest in a pocket-size bottle of eye drops. A final tip: **Avoid getting high in situations where you will need to act like you are not high.** Doing so is a weird waste of weed and can be an exhausting, lightly harrowing pain in the ass. (Exceptions to this rule are funerals and Thanksgiving dinners with extended family.)

KILL STINK FAST WITH A VINEGAR RAG!

Need to get rid of a lingering pot smell as quickly as possible? Proceed directly to the miraculous device known as a vinegar rag, which is exactly what it suggests: a clean rag or dishtowel or promotional T-shirt soaked-but-not-dripping with white vinegar. Once armed with such a rag, walk through your stink-filled space swinging the vinegar rag over your head. For a minute or two after vinegar-ragging, a room will smell faintly of vinegar, then it will smell like nothing. DIY Febreze!

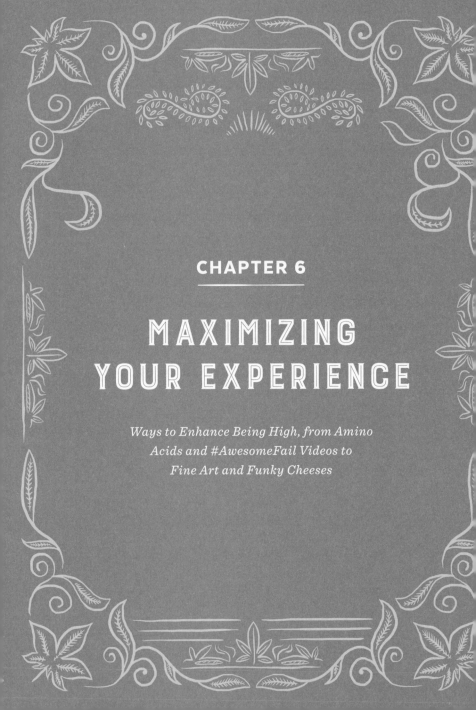

CHAPTER 6

MAXIMIZING YOUR EXPERIENCE

Ways to Enhance Being High, from Amino Acids and #AwesomeFail Videos to Fine Art and Funky Cheeses

ENHANCING THE ACT OF GETTING HIGH

The first step to a good experience with weed is finding a comfortable place to get and be high. By "comfortable," I mean private, secure, and inviting—a reasonably tidied-up living room is perfect. Beyond that, make sure your schedule's clear for a few hours—you don't want to be awaiting phone calls from relatives or visits from cable repairmen.

ENHANCING WEED SMOKING/VAPING: The best way to improve the actual experience of smoking is to do your prep work in advance—de-seed and de-stem your weed, clean your bong/pipe/ashtray, freshen your bong water, prep and clean your vaporizer. Beyond that, have glasses of cool drinking water nearby for potential coughing fits and general refreshment, and think about light scene-setting with music and non-overhead lighting.

BUGGED BY BUTANE? USE A HEMP WICK!

Not into inhaling what comes out of a butane-filled disposable lighter? Get yourself some hemp wicks— inexpensive lengths of lightly waxed hemp twine that hold a slow-burning, butane-free flame for as long as you need.

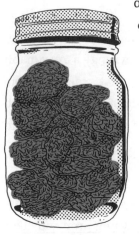

✳ **ENHANCING WEED EATING**: Having a good experience with THC edibles is all about planning and patience. Only a stress-loving doof tries to make cannabis-infused butter, turn that cannabis-infused butter into brownies, then eat those brownies to get high all in the same day. Plan ahead so your day of highness can also be a day of general rest and pleasure (or at least a day of not running around your kitchen monitoring things that are boiling). As I've mentioned, weed that's eaten—and thus processed through the stomach and liver—results in a high that takes up to two hours to hit and can last up to six hours beyond that. So plan ahead to give yourself time to be as patient as edibles

---

WHAT'S THE BEST WAY TO STORE WEED?

Clear ziplock bags are convenient for weed dealers, but aren't the best receptacles for storing weed. To best preserve precious cannabinoids, weed should be stored in an airtight container kept in a cool, dark place. (This cool, dark place can be a refrigerator, but don't put weed buds in a freezer, which can damage the trichomes on the marijuana flowers.) Your best bet is a mason jar with an airtight lid, stashed in a cupboard.

require users to be, and to enjoy your high when it hits. (Aim for a weekend, and don't eat THC edibles too late in the day—ingestion at eight p.m. means high at ten p.m. and for many hours after.)

MAKING THE MOST OF TIME SPENT HIGH

For many people, getting high is synonymous with relaxing and doing whatever the hell one feels like doing. If this is you, you may tell this section to eff off. But if you'd like some tips for making the most of what weed has to offer—from an enhanced ability to marvel at the basic wonders of life to the capacity to fully immerse in tasks like listening to music, raking leaves, and going down on your beloved—here's a guided tour through the primary pleasure centers of the high person's world.

୬ FOOD ୬

Thanks to THC's tweaking of the brain's olfactory center, weed enhances users ability to smell and taste food, making everything from the lowliest corn chip to the swankiest sushi explode with new shades of flavor and a richness of texture that can itself feel intoxicating.

The old joke that stoners love junk food is true—weed can turn a bag of Doritos into a three-act opera in your mouth. But THC is just as effective at enhancing *actual* food, so plan ahead to have the type of food you'd most like to appreciate while high on hand. (Avoid shopping while stoned, which can do ridiculous things to your gastrointestinal system and bank account.) Recommended options: a cheese plate with bread, fruit, and nuts; some luxurious dessert item you rarely allow yourself; ten dollars worth of whatever you want from 7-Eleven.

If you're planning on cooking something, do so before you get high—the combination of stoves and stoned people can go wrong in too many ways. (However, having a puff right before sitting down to a home-cooked meal can be heaven on earth.) If you absolutely have to cook something while high, restrict yourself to the microwave or a slow cooker.

But unless you're some kitchen-loving maniac, you should get high and let someone else feed you. (If this someone is Chef Boyardee, so be it.) Your options are limited only by your preferences and delivery range. Among the classics are delivery pizza, Thai takeout (pick up before you get high or pick a place within walking distance), and walking through the Taco Bell drive-through.

Looking to keep your munchies-based caloric intake in the non-humiliating range? Plan ahead by stocking up lower-calorie foods that can be eaten in excess without much fallout: air-popped popcorn, baked pretzels, chilled grapes, Popsicles.

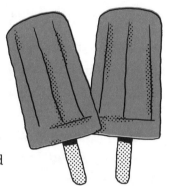

Thinking you might want to try dining out while high? Know that leaving your home severely diminishes your ability to openly discuss being high, aim for somewhere you can walk or bus to, and have a glorious time.

ART AND ENTERTAINMENT

No matter the art form or entertainment genre, weed can enhance your ability to immerse yourself in it, with enriched perception and deeper emotional involvement. (Weed can also leave users—especially new ones—stupefied and unable to follow anything more complex than Teletubbies. See how it goes.) Here are some tips for finding the best match for your high self across the art-and-entertainment spectrum.

Audio/visual entertainments and high folks go together like peanut butter and jelly—perfectly fine on their own, but singularly powerful together. Best bets for high audiences:

🌿 **BRIGHT SHINY COMEDY.** You'll never appreciate a big goofy comedy—*Airplane!, Spaceballs, Borat*—more than when you're high. But THC's powers of comedy enhancement—fueled by immersive focus and general euphoria—extend past the big-and-goofy to every comedy ever made, from edgy cable shows (*South Park, Key & Peele, Broad City*) to beloved sitcoms (*Arrested Development, The Office*) to laugh-out-loud cinema classics (*The Princess Bride, The Big Lebowski, Romy and Michele's High School Reunion*). You cannot go wrong pointing your high eyes at comedy (up to and including *America's Funniest Home Videos*, which has been known to give high people rolling comedy orgasms).

🌿 **SPECIAL-EFFECTS THRILL RIDES.** Dazzle your enhanced synapses with big-bang adventures. THC newbies might want to aim for the plot-driven pleasures of *Star Wars* and *Harry Potter* movies, while more experienced stoners can direct their THC-expanded faculties at the deep-thinking pleasures of *Blade Runner* and *The Matrix*.

🌿 **ANYTHING ANIMATED.** You can go simple (*Scooby-Doo*), you can go artsy (*The Triplets of Belleville*), or you can go nuts (Comedy Central's Adult Swim). But you can't go wrong showing animation to high people. (Truly, it is before an audience of the high that the visual richness and conceptual depth of Pixar films really pay off.)

⭐ **IMMERSIVE DREAMSCAPES.** Among THC's film-enhancing powers is an improved ability to draw connections between disparate images and ideas, which can enrich the hell out of such fill-in-the-blanks dreamscape films like Stanley Kubrick's *2001: A Space Odyssey*, Robert Altman's *3 Women*, and David Lynch's *Mulholland Drive*, while transforming the visually ravishing image parades of films like *Koyaanisqatsi* and *Baraka* into documentaries about the meaning of life.

⭐ **OLD FAVORITES.** Re-watch a movie you've seen previously and loved. This is a great way to highlight how THC can expand perception and intensify focus—you'll be delighted by stuff you previously missed—and since you already know the basic plot, there's little risk of getting lost.

⭐ **STONER GAWKFESTS.** A twisted subgenre of comedy, stoner gawkfests are those perversely comedic works that highlight how gloriously fucked up life can be.

DIVINE IN *PINK FLAMINGOS*

Classics include early John Waters movies (*Pink Flamingos, Female Trouble*), reality shows about other people's problems (*Hoarders, Judge Judy*), and so-bad-they're-good movies like *Road House* and *The Room*. (Advanced-placement gawkfests that should be sought out by aficionados: the TV-clip masterwork *TV Carnage: Casual Fridays*, Jeff Krulik and John Heyn's classic urban-nature short *Heavy Metal Parking Lot*, and Shari Cookson's long-lost, stunningly incisive, thoroughly dark-sided documentary *Living Dolls: The Making of an American Beauty Queen*.)

GET HIGH AND WATCH *SHOWGIRLS*!

Fun fact: I, David Schmader, enjoy getting high and watching the movie *Showgirls* so much that I've done exactly that at cinemas all over the country, with MGM ultimately inviting me to supply my running commentary to the *Showgirls* DVD. For those not familiar, *Showgirls* is Paul Verhoeven's hilariously terrible 1995 stripper drama and I cannot recommend getting high and watching it highly enough. (Skip the rape scene near the end though, which is indefensibly brutal and ruins the hilarious mood.)

MUSIC

Why does getting high enrich one's ability to get rapturously lost in music? A key reason is THC's triggering of the brain's center for auditory stimulation, which allows users to engage more deeply. Some users reporting bouts of synesthesia, wherein visual and auditory senses commingle to create a sense of "seeing" music. But even without audio/visual hallucinations, just the basic act of listening to music while high can be deeply rewarding. If you're looking for foolproof stoner-pleasing albums, you cannot go wrong with Brian Eno's soundscape-with-songs *Another Green World,* Clifford Brown's jazz ravishment *With Strings*, Tricky's trip-hop masterwork *Maxinquaye*, the Beatles' "White Album," or the collected works of Bob Marley.

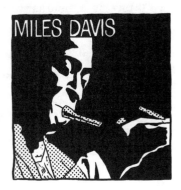

(Also, D'Angelo's *Voodoo*, Van Morrison's *Moondance,* Miles Davis's *Kind of Blue* and *In a Silent Way*, DJ Shadow's *Endtroducing*....., the Grateful Dead's *American Beauty,* and the self-titled third album by the Velvet Underground.)

VISUAL ART

From dramatic Rothko color-fields to towering Serra sculptures to brain-spiking Holzer slogans, visual art can be highly rewarding for high people. Part of this is THC's expansion of the senses, which allows users to engage with art more deeply—seeing a painting as a conversation, plugging into the thousand and one choices that go into the creation of a work, softly weeping at a particular shade of pale green. So at least once in your life, point your high eyes at some art. If there's a museum you can walk or bus to (and you feel comfortable being high in public), go there and choose your own adventure. (There are two basic options: go deep, falling fully into every piece and losing an entire day, or wear earbuds, playing your favorite music as you stroll about, turning the museum's collection into a spontaneously curated music video.)

But even stoners stranded on sofas can expose themselves to art, via coffee table books or college textbooks or

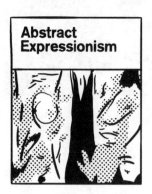

the Internet. Many museums have gorgeous, art-packed websites, or you can just plug artists' names into Google image search. (Some terms to get you started: "Martini Annunciation," "Renoir boating party," and "Georgia O'Keefe vagina flower.")

VIDEO GAMES

According to people who enjoy both weed and competitive virtual realities, there are few things more fun than getting high and playing video games. Chalk this up to THC's enhancement of audio/visual stimulation and high people's improved immersion skills, with weed causing the real world to recede, leaving high gamers locked in battle with their *Minecrafts* and *Grand Theft Autos* and *Alien: Defenestrations*. (If you're not a gamer and would like to have your mind blown, get high and have a knowledgeable friend give you a guided tour of a twenty-first-century video game. The future is now, and insane.)

GO EXPLORING

For some, leaving the house while high is an invitation to be bombarded by a million paranoia triggers. For others, it's the most natural thing in the world. If you're the second sort, here are some suggested targets for exploration.

✴ **YOUR CITY.** Go wherever your feet and/or public transportation can take you. Aim for your city's delightful parts: parks, sculpture gardens, public markets, waterfront boardwalks. (But even a stroll around the neighborhood can be an experiential adventure.)

✦ **THE NATURAL WORLD.** Exploring nature while high can be as simple as finding a sunny patch of grass on a lawn or as complicated as snowshoeing over a mountain. What matters is getting your high self out in nature. Get lost in an arboretum. Wade in a lake. Take a blanket out at night and look at the stars. When high folks behold nature, they find as much delight as they're willing to look for.

✦ **THE WORLD WIDE WEB.** Opened to the simplest web browser, any computer can be a portal to a vast virtual wilderness packed with more delights that you can conceive. Don't believe me? Google anything. Google something you love—a band or artist or TV show or historical period. Or just Google random stuff—"chimps doing plays" and "wet wigs" and "wedding bloopers." (If there's anything that might make Chatroulette non-prohibitively squirm-inducing, it's weed.)

GET CREATIVE

From the films of Robert Altman to the music of Cypress Hill to the comedy of Sarah Silverman, weed's ability to inspire and enhance creativity is well documented. Get in on the act by steering your high self toward a creative endeavor. Drawing, painting, taking photos, creating GIFs—virtually any creative act that's worth doing is worth doing high (at least once). Aim for unrestricted creative endeavors: Weed can be highly inspirational for brainstorming and freewriting, but don't get high to write a final draft. You'll need input from your non-high brain for that.

GET SEXUAL

With its enhancement of the senses, expansion of perception, and intensification of focus, weed can make sex an astoundingly intoxicating and gratifying act. Just kissing can feel deeply sexual, and exploration below the neck can feel like a trip around the world. Still, weed's sex-enhancing effects depend entirely on the person and the weed, with some high people made so introspective or cerebral that sex is off the menu. Best bet for sexy times: a nice indica-dominant hybrid, which gets you in your body without anchoring you to the sofa. (Flying solo? High masturbation can be killer too.)

ASSORTED OTHER STUFF
✺ THAT CAN BE FUN TO DO HIGH ✺

✻ **HOUSE/YARD WORK.** Gather your tools and supplies, put on music you love, and watch your domestic to-do list melt in a haze of pleasingly repetitive movement and singing along.

✻ **TAKING A BATH.** First, get high, put on a podcast, and clean your bathtub. Then strip naked and show that bathtub what it's made for. Water and high folks are a magical combination. (Even a shower can feel like a mini-vacation.)

✳ **HANGING OUT WITH DOGS.** Have a dog? Grab your fetching balls and poop bags and get to it. Don't have a dog? Go to a dog park. Just watching other people's dogs be dogs can be extraordinarily entertaining. (Caution: Do not go to a dog shelter high. Dog adoption is serious business, and you should go when you're not in empathy drenched sensualist escape mode.)

ENHANCING THE EFFECTS OF THC

Attain your highest high with these weed hacks.

✳ **TAKE A BREAK.** Regular weed smoking naturally builds up a user's tolerance to THC, so if you're looking to attain peak highness, take regular breaks from weed. Going a few days (or a few weeks) without smoking helps clear your cannabinoid receptors and lets you feel way more of your high.

✳ **MIX UP YOUR METHODS.** Always use a bong? Try a vaporizer! Always smoke a certain strain? Try another! Our cannabinoid receptors habituate to whatever THC delivery system we use most, so throw 'em a curve ball once in a while and reap the rewards of a new type of high.

✳ EAT MANGOES. According to stoner lore, eating a mango forty-five minutes to an hour before getting high can significantly enhance the experience, thanks to the chemical compound myrcene, which is found in both mangos and marijuana and speeds the delivery of THC to the brain. (Other vitamins and supplements that allegedly amp the effects of THC include omega-3 fatty acids and vitamin C.)

DOES HOLDING SMOKE IN AND/ OR COUGHING GET YOU HIGHER?

According to stoner lore, weed smokers can amplify their highs by holding smoke in their lungs for an extended period of time and coughing afterward. Regarding holding smoke in, studies suggest 85 to 95 percent of THC is absorbed within seconds of inhalation, with the key "benefits" of extended smoke-holding being a larger tar deposit on the lungs and a bit of a head rush caused by oxygen deprivation. As for coughing, lore posits that violent hacking makes your lungs expand, thus increasing the surface area of your lungs exposed to THC-spiked smoke. However, this theory remains something someone's cousin told them once, and the main "benefits" of violent coughing seem to be an oxygen-deprivation head rush.

CHAPTER 7

IF YOU'RE HIGH 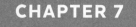 DON'T LIKE IT

Navigating the Murky and Worse
Sides of Highness

I n the history of the world, there is no record of a fatal marijuana overdose. Nevertheless, many people have gotten so high that they wish they were dead, which is terrifying. Beyond psychic meltdowns, many other people have gotten high and simply not liked it, with all the expected feelings of euphoria and sensual enhancement eclipsed by panic and paranoia and a racing heart rate. Should you ever find yourself in the grip of an unpleasant marijuana high, follow these tips.

★ **RELAX.** Remember how I said no one's ever died from getting too high? It's true, and you should ruminate on that fact as you take at least three deep breaths, slowly in and slowly out. You're going to be fine; you just need to be patient and take care of yourself as you ride out your unpleasant but not dangerous high.

★ **SQUEEZE A LEMON.** One of the few things known to diminish extreme highness is limonene, a terpene that modulates THC's effects on the brain and is conveniently found in lemons. Should you find yourself too high for your taste, squeeze juice from a fresh lemon, zest in a bit of peel, add as much sugar as necessary, and toss the whole thing down your throat. According to science, it should help.

🌿 **SMELL SOME PEPPER.** Another terpene-based maneuver, this one involves beta-caryophyllene, a terpene found in 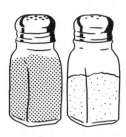 black pepper that's specifically cited for its ability to combat weed-based paranoia. To activate it, smash or grind a few fresh peppercorns, then get your nose down close and take a big whiff. Sneeze afterward if you must.

🌿 **BE NICE TO YOURSELF.** Remind yourself that you're in no danger and the state you're in is temporary. Surround yourself with stuff that makes you feel safe. (If this means pajamas in bed, so be it.) Don't fixate on your inability to think straight or berate yourself over a word you can't remember— steer yourself toward things that make you feel secure.

🌿 **TAKE A COLD SHOWER.** This probably won't feel so much like "being nice to yourself," but there's no denying the power of a cold shower to reboot a nervous system.

🌿 **GET SOME FRESH AIR.** Deep breaths are good, and deep breaths of fresh air are better. If you're not up for taking a walk, open a window.

🌿 **EAT SOMETHING.** Aim for something substantial and nutritious: yogurt, fresh fruit, microwaved soup, healthy cereal.

✴ **DRINK WATER.** Not only does it keep you hydrated, it helps flush your system.

✴ **TALK TO SOMEONE.** Have a trusted friend who's familiar with weed? Sharing your too-high experience with someone who understands can help a ton. Ask for what you need, up to and including, "I need you to call me every forty-five minutes to remind me that I'm fine until I tell you to stop."

✴ **REST.** Lie down. Close your eyes. Get comfortable. Whether or not you actually doze is immaterial—just restricting your world to your bed/couch and the backs of your eyelids helps. Take deep breaths, following each breath in and each breath out.

Along with the "dos" come some "don'ts": Don't answer the phone unless you know who's calling and want to talk. Don't use a stove or drive a car. Don't stare at yourself in a mirror or give yourself a haircut. And when your bad bout of highness is over, don't neglect to Google "Maureen Dowd Colorado" to confirm how not alone you are.

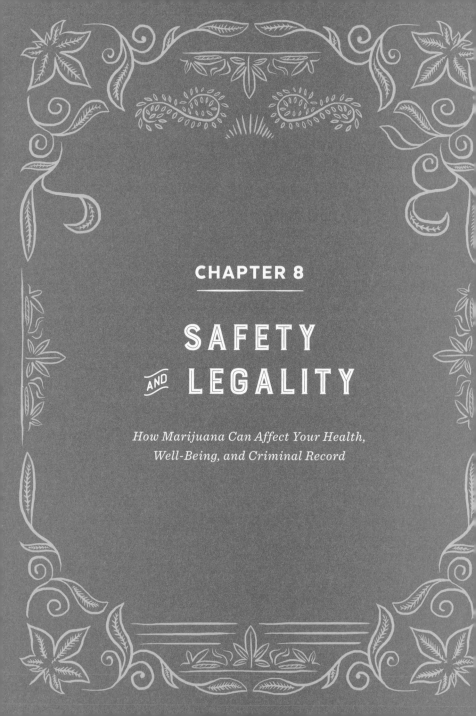

CHAPTER 8

SAFETY & LEGALITY

How Marijuana Can Affect Your Health,
Well-Being, and Criminal Record

Despite its pleasures and benefits, weed is not entirely safe and, unless you live in one of the blessed states with modified laws, it's the opposite of legal. Getting caught with weed in a prohibition state can seriously mess up your life—cost you jobs, complicate your housing options, get you rejected for organ transplants—and even the most careful use in any state invites potential risks to your health and well-being.

WEED SAFETY

On the list of dangerous drugs, marijuana ranks near the bottom, primarily because it's all but impossible to ingest a lethal dose of weed. (Even aspirin can kill you if you take too much, but a fatal dose of marijuana would require ingestion of fifteen hundred pounds in fifteen minutes—a physical impossibility for any human, even Snoop Dogg.)

But just because it's not deadly doesn't mean it's safe. THC is a powerful intoxicant that can impair physical ability and judgment in ways that could get you hurt or killed. And heavy use of marijuana can lead to an array of problems, most notably for users under the age of eighteen. (See Kids and Weed: Two Great Things That Should Be Kept Far, Far Apart on page 155.)

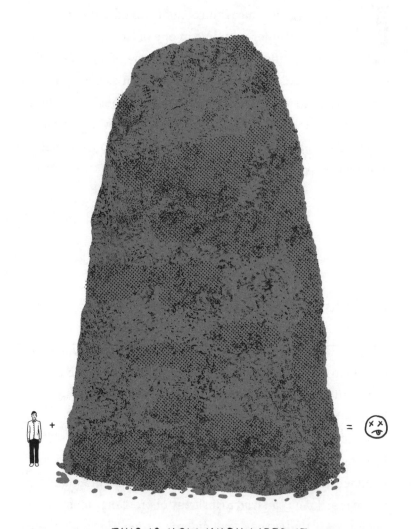

THIS IS HOW MUCH WEED IT
WOULD TAKE TO KILL YOU.

⌒ ADDICTION RISKS ⌒

The standard claim is that marijuana is not physically addictive, because unlike opiates such as heroin, weed doesn't saddle users with desperate physical cravings or leave them physically wrecked during withdrawals. Nevertheless, habitual use of marijuana can absolutely create psychological dependence, with users coming to rely on weed to relax or be creative or just get to sleep. And while weed withdrawal symptoms fall short of the vomity horrors of heroin, they're still no picnic, with heavy weed users who quit (or run out) reporting seriously unpleasant symptoms—insomnia, headaches, night sweats, concentration problems, hair-trigger mood swings, freaky dreams—that can last from a week to a month or more.

So how does one avoid becoming the type of heavy habitual weed user whose life sucks when weed is removed from the equation? It's tempting to suggest the same rules used for responsible drinking (only after five p.m. or on weekends, never alone, no driving). But weed comes with its own specific temptations, especially for users who appreciate the relaxation, focus, and bursts of creativity THC can bestow, and may consider such beneficial effects as justification for more regular use.

Nevertheless, for all weed users, the "treat it like booze!" mandate is a solid guideline. If you have a puff when you get home from work (and this post-work puff doesn't lead to an evening of endless follow-up puffs), you'll likely be fine. If your weed use continues despite negative consequences— relationship problems, memory problems, money problems— know that you're on the path to a weirdly restricted life and, eventually, crappy withdrawals. If you need help quitting weed, visit Marijuana Anonymous online: Marijuana-Anonymous.org. (Regarding claims of "skyrocketing" rates of marijuana addiction, there's no divorcing such claims from the many arrested potheads who are offered a stint in rehab over a stint in jail, with many "treatment-seeking addicts" just unlucky weed appreciators looking to avoid the slammer.)

IS WEED A "GATEWAY DRUG"?

A "gateway drug" is an intoxicant that inspires users to try other, scarier intoxicants: smoke weed on a Monday, the gateway theorists contend, and you'll be freebasing cocaine by Friday. But the fact is that the majority of marijuana's potential as a gateway drug comes from its prohibition, which forces users to engage with the black market, often through dealers with way more to sell than weed and incentive to sell as much of everything as possible. So yes, buying illegal weed can put users within the orbit of other illegal drugs. But it's not the weed's fault.

৬ CANCER ৬

In the early 2000s, UCLA researchers conducted a comprehensive study of the cancer risks of smoking cannabis, and were surprised to find that smoking weed—even heavy, regular weed smoking—doesn't lead to lung cancer, throat cancer, or any other type of head/neck cancer. There are still plenty of reasons to avoid smoking weed, but as of now, cancer isn't one of them. (For information on how marijuana can actually help those with cancer, see Chapter 9: Medical Marijuana 101.)

৬ CARDIOVASCULAR CONCERNS ৬

Immediately after smoking, users will experience dilated blood vessels and an elevated heart rate, which can be scary and potentially hazardous for those with preexisting heart conditions. The fact is that everyone who smokes marijuana—whether they have preexisting heart conditions or not—is five times more likely to have a heart attack within the first hour of smoking than someone who's smoked nothing. This is alarming until you realize this is commensurate with the heart-attack risks of having sex and jogging. If you have a history of heart trouble, or even a history of worrying that you might have heart trouble, smoking weed is not for you.

৶ COGNITIVE IMPAIRMENT ৶

Marijuana temporarily impairs a number of mental functions, with high people having difficulty remembering details, following conversations, and performing complex tasks. The good news is that these difficulties last only as long as the high—once users sober up, their brain function should be back to normal (though some users report sluggish-brain hangovers the day after). Even chronic users appear to be at low risk for permanent neuropsychological complications. (The great exception is users under the age of eighteen. See Kids and Weed: Two Great Things That Should Be Kept Far, Far Apart on page 155.)

৶ PSYCHOLOGICAL RISKS ৶

From panic attacks to temporary psychosis to depression, THC can cause an array of unpleasant psycho-emotional effects. If weed makes you panicky or depressed, congratulations. You now have concrete evidence that weed is not for you and are free to live the rest of your life waving off bongs and spiked brownies without compunction. On a more serious note, recent years have brought attention to the possible link between marijuana and schizophrenia, but the existing links seem to be genetic (if you have a family history of schizophrenia, marijuana might precipitate it) and most specifically concern young users with still-developing brains.

For the vast majority of the population, adult weed use does not lead to increased rates of mental illness.

PSYCHOMOTOR
⤳ PERFORMANCE IMPAIRMENT ⤶

THC can seriously impair psychomotor function, especially for new users, who can be waylaid by loss of coordination, impaired distance perception, and erratic reaction times. This is why driving while high is not only illegal but idiotic. No sane stoned person *wants* to drive, but sometimes someone tries to talk you into it (and sometimes this someone is yourself). Whatever the case, don't do it. To quote that diabolical wigstand Nancy Reagan, "Just Say No."

⤳ PULMONARY/RESPIRATORY RISKS ⤶

People who smoke weed all the time are very likely to experience symptoms of bronchitis, including chronic cough and an increase in respiratory infections. But moderate users (up to and including those who smoke a joint a day) have been found to have no diminishment of lung function, and even in the heaviest weed smokers there's no increased rate of obstructive pulmonary disease (a standard affliction for cigarette smokers). As always, if you want to avoid problems associated with smoking, get a vaporizer.

॰ REPRODUCTIVE HEALTH RISKS ॰

Studies suggest heavy marijuana use might complicate reproduction for both sexes, reducing fertility in women and lowering sperm counts in men. If you are actively striving to conceive, lay off the weed. Does weed lead to birth defects? No studies have confirmed a risk, but not many studies have been undertaken, and every sane female pothead I know has given up weed the second she learned she was pregnant. (A number of them also enjoyed large, congratulatory bong hits once they stopped breastfeeding.)

As for dudes, there's no hard evidence that weed can lead to infertility, and the aforementioned drop in sperm production is temporary, with counts returning to normal once a guy stops regular weed use. The big male concern remain "moobs"—"man boobs" allegedly created by overindulgence in weed, which can cause testosterone levels to drop, inspiring estrogen levels to rise to cover the spread, and leaving male potheads with puffy little bosoms. This moob-creating hormonal-imbalance situation is real—doctors call it "gynecomastia"—and its connection to weed is not yet concrete but probable for regular heavy users.

So if you're a guy who abhors the idea of an enhanced bust line, don't smoke tons of weed.

KIDS AND WEED: TWO GREAT THINGS THAT SHOULD BE KEPT FAR, FAR APART

You know those previously mentioned risks involving body-morphing hormonal imbalances and elevated potential for schizophrenia? They're even riskier for weed users under the age of eighteen, whose brains and bodies are still developing and are weirdly susceptible to the worst things THC can do. Heavy marijuana use during puberty and adolescence is a reliable path to a seriously troubled life, with heavy users hobbled by slower brains, diminished learning capacities, and a heightened susceptibility for mental illness, from panic attacks to schizophrenia. Humans under the age of eighteen should not smoke or otherwise imbibe marijuana.

WEED LEGALITY

Marijuana is illegal in the United States, where it's classified alongside heroin and LSD as a Schedule 1 drug with high potential for abuse and no established medical use. The use, possession, sale, cultivation, and transportation of marijuana is illegal under federal law in the United States of America.

However, a growing number of states within the United States are rescinding, declawing, or otherwise modifying their marijuana laws, creating a nation where weed is illegal, full of states where weed is maybe not illegal. This odd arrangement is made possible through a semiformal truce between the federal government and the states, with the feds acknowledging a state's right to decriminalize weed for medical or recreational use, and states acknowledging the feds' good sportsmanship by establishing regulation systems and other totems of responsible social integration around their decriminalized weed.

At the time of this writing, marijuana is fully legal for medicinal and recreational use in four states (Colorado, Washington, Alaska, and Oregon) and two cities (Portland and South Portland in Maine). It's also legal for medicinal and recreational use in the District of Columbia, but retail sales have thus far been blocked by Congress.

Eleven more states have legal medical marijuana and decriminalized recreational marijuana. (Decriminalization doesn't make weed legal, it just makes possession of small amounts a minor infraction on par with a traffic ticket.) Nine more states plus Guam have legalized weed for medical use only, while three states plus the US Virgin Islands have decriminalized weed without establishing specific laws around medical use. As you can tell, things are in flux, but here are some basic facts to help you along.

IS THERE WEIRD STUFF IN MY WEED?

It's nice to imagine that all marijuana is grown by generous-spirited hippies adhering to organic ideals. Unfortunately, this isn't the case. While tracking THC levels in black-market weed, researchers also encountered many contaminants, from pesticides and heavy metals to mold and bacteria. Is weed cleaner in states where it's legal? Yes. For example, Washington State tests its legal recreational weed for E. coli, salmonella, and mold—and 13 percent of weed products offered for sale in 2014 were rejected as tainted. If you're in a prohibition state, find a dealer you trust and hope for the best. (And if you ever get a chance to vote on legalizing marijuana, vote yes.)

৩ MEDICAL MARIJUANA ৬

In states with legal medical weed, people typically become medical marijuana patients by visiting a doctor who listens to their symptoms and deems them worthy of a written certification recommending medical marijuana. (Under federal law, doctors can't *prescribe* weed, but thanks to the First Amendment, they can *recommend* it.) Among the most common symptoms and afflictions treated with medical marijuana are nausea, gastrointestinal disorders, insomnia, and menstrual cramps. For a thorough list of marijuana's medical uses, see Chapter 9: Medical Marijuana 101.

Can someone with medical marijuana legally travel with their medicine to another state? If the destination state also has legal medical weed, it should be no problem, and traveling patients should check to see if the involved states have reciprocity laws, which allow one state's medical marijuana patients to acquire medicine in another state. But if a patient is traveling to a state that hasn't legalized medical marijuana, his or her medicine reverts back to contraband the minute they cross the state line. In prohibition states, medical marijuana patients can be charged with possession, and if they've transported their medicine over state lines, they could face federal charges for drug trafficking.

WHERE'S THE BEST PLACE TO SMOKE WEED IN A PROHIBITION STATE?

You should smoke in the most private part of your private residence. Pick a room as far as possible from the front door—you don't want the smell detectable to everyone who comes knocking. Contain your stink as best you can. Smoking by open windows makes sense in post-prohibition states, but doing so where weed's illegal can release a scent that adds up to reasonable suspicion for police to search your place. If you can afford it, get one of those Ionic Breeze air purifiers. Otherwise, school yourself on the miraculous power of the vinegar rag, explicated on page 125.

As for flying with medical marijuana, airports are federal jurisdictions, and patients can be busted while going through security. The feds don't care about medical marijuana authorizations from any state.

⤸ RECREATIONAL MARIJUANA ⤿

In prohibition states, a first-offense, personal-use marijuana possession charge is typically a misdemeanor but can rise to the level of felony through a variety of factors, including prior arrests, being busted near a school or designated community center, or being caught in connection with a driving infraction. Penalties for marijuana possession can include mandatory drug testing, a suspended driver's license, fines of up to two thousand dollars, and even jail time. (Typically less than a year, but still.) If you're busted for possession of marijuana, get yourself a lawyer immediately.

↞ WEED AND DRUG TESTS ↠

Thanks to being stored in the body's fat cells, THC takes longer to leave the body than most drugs. It's hard to determine exactly how long THC hangs around, as everybody's metabolism is different. But the general guideline suggests that one-time weed use leaves detectable evidence in blood for twelve to twenty-four hours and in urine for one to seven days, while regular use leaves detectable evidence in blood for two to seven days and in urine from one week to three months. It's important to note that urine tests don't detect the psychoactive THC, but the non-psychoactive marijuana compound THC-COOH, which can linger in the body for days and weeks after smoking, making urine tests good for detecting prior weed use but ineffectual at determining real-time highness. For that, blood tests are needed, and they are typically used in connection with investigations of DUIs and workplace injuries.

Scheduled to take a drug test and worried about **weed in** your system? The Internet offers a buttload of allegedly **help-**ful suggestions, from "consume a half-dozen energy **drinks** as fast as possible" to "acquire clean pee." Investigate **at your** own risk.

HOW LONG DOES THC STAY IN YOUR SYSTEM?

	ONE-TIME USE	**REGULAR USE**
BLOOD	12 to 24 hours	2 to 7 days
URINE	1 to 7 days	1 week to 3 months

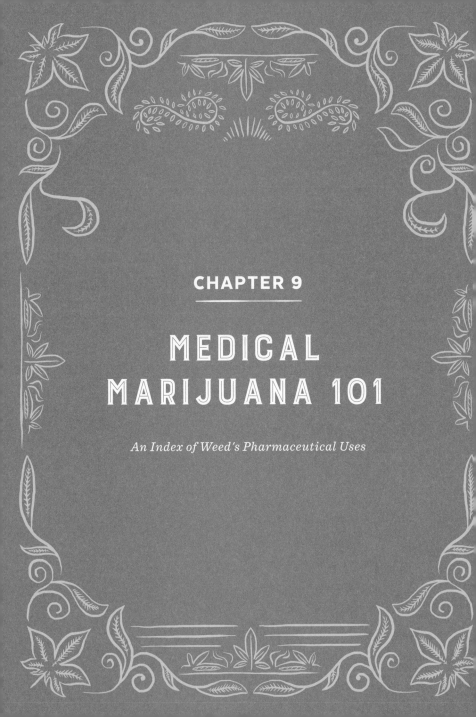

CHAPTER 9

MEDICAL MARIJUANA 101

An Index of Weed's Pharmaceutical Uses

Marijuana has been used as medicine for thousands of years. Typically, weed has been used not as an active treatment for disease, but for its palliative effects, which reliably diminish symptoms and side effects of AIDS, cancer, Crohn's disease, epilepsy, multiple sclerosis, and arthritis, and have recently shown promise in treating psychological disorders like PTSD.

The medical use of marijuana was carried out without much fanfare until the start of the twentieth century, when the many cannabis-infused medicines on American drugstore shelves were subject to a permanent recall, thanks to the anti-marijuana bias enshrined in law by Harry Anslinger's Marihuana Tax Act of 1937. Restrictions were further enhanced by the Controlled Substances Act of 1970, which placed marijuana among Schedule 1 drugs, a classification reserved for substances with a high potential for abuse and no recognized medicinal use.

This Schedule 1 classification is the greatest obstacle to marijuana-related sanity in the United States. Consider the Schedule 1 specification of "no recognized medical use": With all of weed's well-documented palliative effects, isn't this designation demonstrably false? You'd think so, but the studies that would officially confirm marijuana's stature as medicine have been stymied by marijuana's stature as a restricted Schedule 1 drug.

CBD: THE CANNABINOID WITH TONS OF MEDICAL POTENTIAL AND ZERO PSYCHOACTIVE SIDE EFFECTS

Forever working against the recognition of marijuana as medicine is its ability to get users pleasantly high, which, in the minds of reactionary nimrods, makes all support for medical marijuana tainted by drug-seeking motives. This is one of a million reasons to cherish **cannabidiol**, popularly abbreviated to CBD. Unlike the popular THC, CBD has zero psychoactive effects, giving users access to weed's medical benefits without requiring them to get stoned. Marijuana breeders are now creating strains with high levels of CBD and almost no THC, opening medical marijuana treatment possibilities for many patients who don't want to get high—for example, children with seizure disorders.

THC	CBD
Gets you high	Does not get you high
Increases appetite	Increases appetite
Decreases nausea	Decreases nausea
Relieves pain	Relieves pain
Inspires euphoria	Decreases seizures, spasms, and convulsions
	Reduces inflammation and anxiety

For example, to do clinical research of Schedule 2 drugs like cocaine and methamphetamine, researchers need only to whip up their desired substance in a lab. But for a fiercely restricted Schedule 1 drug like marijuana, researchers need to jump through hoops not demanded of drugs with lower classifications, including getting licensed by the Drug Enforcement Agency (DEA) to legally handle the contraband, having their studies preapproved by the Food and Drug Administration (FDA), and being granted research-grade marijuana from the National Institute on Drug Abuse (NIDA), whose official mission is to research the harmful effects of controlled substances and has little interest in researching weed's non-harmful benefits.

Then there's the issue of money, and the difficulty of acquiring funding for marijuana research. Typically a good portion of such funding comes from pharmaceutical companies, which are eager to find the next patentable-and-marketable drug. But there's no patenting a plant that grows everywhere, and with diminished hopes of profit, marijuana research is left to lag. (Besides being un-patentable, medical marijuana might feasibly serve as an alternative to existing patented drugs, making marijuana research doubly unattractive to pharmacological profit seekers, while fueling theories that weed's Schedule 1 designation is in part a sop to Big Pharma.)

Nevertheless, professional pharmacology has managed to patent two marijuana-derived drugs approved for use in the United States: Dronabinol, a synthetic cannabinoid recommended as a treatment for nausea and vomiting in AIDS and cancer patients, and Nabilone, another synthetic cannabinoid used to treat nausea and vomiting that's also shown promise in treating neuropathic pain, with one study showing patients who combined their existing pain medication with Nabilone experienced pain reduction of 30 percent or more, with minimal side effects. Still, the isolated synthetic cannabinoids in both Dronabinol and Nabilone have been found to be less effective, with worse side effects, than the harmonious bundle of cannabinoids found in marijuana.

If/when marijuana is finally moved from the highly restrictive Schedule 1 classification to the medical research-enabling

Schedule 2 or lower, the cumulative knowledge around weed's medicinal benefits will firm up, gain authority, and very likely expand in all directions. For now, here's a list of ailments most frequently treated with medical marijuana. (Potential side effects of all medical marijuana use: increased heart rate, decreased blood pressure, dizziness/lightheadedness, dry mouth, short-term memory inhibition, and general stonedness.)

✶ **AIDS/HIV.** Among the many life-imperiling illnesses that may visit people with AIDS is wasting syndrome—acute malnutrition that allows fat and muscle tissue to dissolve. During the height of the 1980s AIDS crisis, many potentially fatal bouts of wasting syndrome were survived with the help of medical marijuana, which enhanced appetites and diminished nausea of patients previously unable to eat to literally save their lives. (See the glossary entry for Brownie Mary on page 174.) Beyond wasting, weed can minimize the nausea that can accompany lifesaving HIV medications and has helped countless AIDS patients eat, sleep, and experience diminished pain.

✶ **ANOREXIA.** Thanks to THC's triggering of cannabinoid receptors that increase hunger and decrease nausea, marijuana can be an effective treatment for anorexia patients and others suffering illness-induced appetite suppression.

✶ **ARTHRITIS.** The primary compounds of weed, THC and CBD, have shown promise in diminishing the pain of arthritis, thanks to cannabinoids' analgesic effects and anti-inflammatory properties, which can diminish pain while reducing the inflammation that caused the pain in the first place.

✶ **CANCER.** Marijuana has long been known to combat nausea caused by chemotherapy while enhancing appetites of chemo-clobbered patients. But there's growing curiosity about weed's potential as a weapon against cancer itself, with evidence suggesting marijuana extracts may impede cancer growth, improve the effects of radiation treatment, and even kill cancer cells with minimal damage to surrounding cells.

✶ **CHRONIC PAIN.** Unlike opiates, cannabinoids don't block pain, they just decrease the number of pain messages sent from the nerves to the brain, producing a reliable analgesic effect that's helped sufferers of fibromyalgia, arthritis, and migraine manage their pain and decrease their dependence on liver-taxing opiates.

✶ **FIBROMYALGIA.** See Chronic Pain.

✶ **GASTROINTESTINAL ILLNESS.** Smoking marijuana has several promising benefits for sufferers of inflammatory bowel diseases like ulcerative colitis and Crohn's—easing pain, diminishing diarrhea, and aiding weight gain.

🌿 **GLAUCOMA.** It's the go-to ailment for medical marijuana punch lines, but glaucoma is a serious disease of the optic nerve that can result in blindness, and its treatment with marijuana is controversial: weed can lower eye pressure, but it also lowers blood pressure, creating a reduced blood flow that could harm the optic nerve. Proceed with caution.

🌿 **MENSTRUAL CRAMPS.** Weed has been used to ease menstrual discomfort since at least the nineteenth century, when the physician to Queen Victoria prescribed tincture of cannabis to minimize Her Royal Highness's cramps. As many twenty-first-century women can attest, it still works.

HER ROYAL HIGHNESS QUEEN VICTORIA

🌿 **NEUROLOGICAL DISORDERS.** For sufferers of neurological disorders—ALS, epilepsy, multiple sclerosis, Parkinson's disease—marijuana can reduce problematic inflammation, with cannabinoids correcting imbalances in the endocannabinoid system that coincide with neurological degeneration. Specifically, weed has been cited as a treatment for the pain and spasticity of ALS/Lou Gehrig's disease, for the muscle spasms and tremors of multiple sclerosis, and for seizures related to epilepsy.

🌿 **POST-TRAUMATIC STRESS DISORDER (PTSD).** Weed can help PTSD sufferers with insomnia and anxiety, and has also shown promise on the deeper level of memory extinction, which is the natural process of shedding associations from stimuli. (Without memory extinction, we'd be paralyzed by memories of every face we've ever seen.) By helping with memory extinction, marijuana can help PTSD patients reduce associations between real-world stimuli (stress, loud noises) and past trauma.

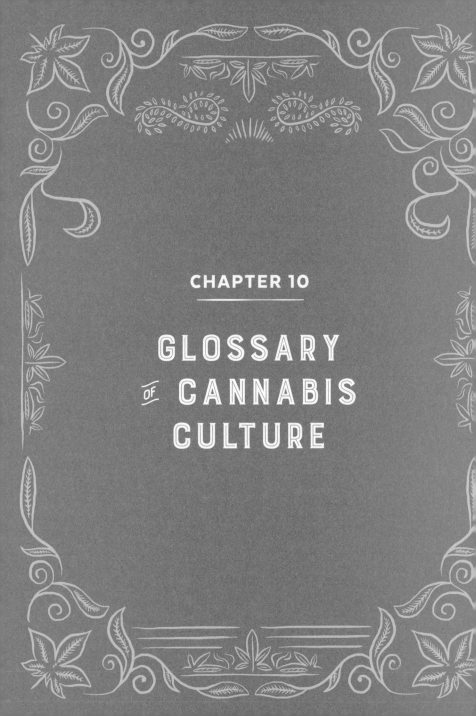

CHAPTER 10

GLOSSARY
of CANNABIS
CULTURE

420: Pronounced "four-twenty," 420 is a multipurpose referent for marijuana, simultaneously used to denote the unofficial "marijuana holiday" on the twentieth of April (4/20), the twice-daily "marijuana time" (4:20 a.m./p.m.), and as a euphemism for marijuana itself: "Got 420?" Lore on the origin of the term abounds, positing everything from 420 being police code for weed busts to being the number of chemical compounds in cannabis. (Neither is true.) The most widely recognized origin story involves a group of friends in Northern California in the early 1970s, who would meet up after school for weed-based adventures at 4:20 p.m. The "420" euphemism was soon picked up by the group's wider circle of friends, which happened to include members of the Grateful Dead, who popularized the term among its fans.

AMERICANS FOR SAFE ACCESS: A member-powered organization founded in 2002 to fight for safe, legal access to medical marijuana. The group's motivating principle is safe access to medical cannabis is a human right.

BOGARTING: A slang term derived from the onscreen persona of film actor Humphrey Bogart, who made a habit of holding a lit cigarette between his fingers and/or his lips, allowing smoke to rise dramatically. "Bogarting a joint" means holding on to it instead of passing it to the next puffer, and typically involves a high person getting so involved in telling a story that they forget about the burning joint in their hand.

BONG WATER: The water held in the bottom of a bong, which cools smoke before it's inhaled, and quickly becomes disgusting as it grows sludgy with ash. Sludgy bong water is easily among the ten grossest-smelling things a normal person will encounter, so protect yourself by changing your bong water frequently (pouring it down the toilet, not the sink, because that stuff's gross). Should you spill ripe, sludgy bong water on your couch or carpet, woe be unto you.

BROWNIE MARY: Nickname of Mary Jane Rathbun, a volunteer at San Francisco General Hospital, who supplied THC brownies to sick and dying patients during the height of the 1980s AIDS crisis. Rathbun made her "magic brownies"—which had lifesaving benefits for patients with wasting syndrome—in her apartment using marijuana donated by sympathetic growers, and distributed her wares free of charge. She was arrested three times, but never stopped campaigning for medical marijuana, eventually helping California to become the first state in the nation to legalize medical weed in 1996.

CANNABIS ACTION NETWORK: A national network of individuals and organizations founded in 1989 to advocate for legal medicinal, industrial, and recreational cannabis and empower those citizens ready to join the fight.

CANNABIS CUP: The world's premiere marijuana trade show, sponsored by *High Times* magazine and held annually in states with legal weed. Among the delights: instructional seminars, product showcases, music performances, and strain competitions.

CANNABIS STRAINS: Pure or hybrid cannabis varieties bred to highlight specific characteristics and effects, and typically given names inspired by a strain's taste, color, smell, or geographical birthplace. (Panama Red, Maui Wowie, White Widow.)

CASHED: Slang for the state of a bong or pipe whose contents have been reduced to ash: "This bowl is cashed."

CHARLOTTE'S WEB: Along with an eternally heart-crushing book by E. B. White, "Charlotte's Web" is the name of a special strain of marijuana that's bred to have high levels of cannabidiol (CBD) and low levels of THC, providing the benefits of medical weed without the high-making effects of THC. Produced by Colorado's Realm of Caring Foundation, the strain is named for Charlotte Figi, an American girl whose chronic seizures were significantly reduced after ingesting an extract of the high-CBD weed.

CHEECH & CHONG: Legendary stoner comedy duo consisting of Richard "Cheech" Marin and Tommy Chong, who became stars in the '70s and '80s with comedy albums and films like 1978's *Up in Smoke*. Their best-remembered contribution to American culture: the 1971 skit "Dave," the de facto "Who's on First?" of stoner comedy, built around the refrain "Dave's not here."

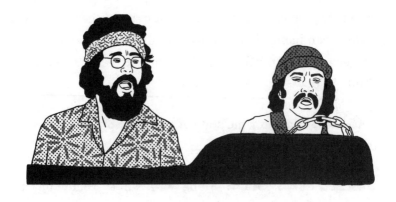

CHERRY: Slang for a chunk of weed in a bong or pipe bowl that stays lit, typically occurring only with tightly packed bowls and/or bud dense enough to hold the burn without flaming out.

THE CHRONIC: The debut solo album of former NWA member Dr. Dre, released in 1992 and taking its name from a strain of red-haired, hyper-powerful weed with its compact disc emblazoned with a large marijuana leaf. Exceedingly popular and expertly produced, *The Chronic* is considered by many to be prime stoner music, while many others are repelled by the violent misogyny and general shitheadedness of the lyrics.

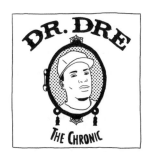

CONTACT HIGH: A psychological phenomenon wherein sober people placed in close proximity to high people ambiently absorb a state of intoxication. (Not to be confused with getting high as the result of inhaling secondhand smoke, which is its own thing.) Are contact highs verifiable occurrences or optimism-fueled placebos? Yes.

COTTONMOUTH: Slang for the state of being that occurs as THC disrupts neural messages to the salivary glands, leaving high people with mouths so dry it's like they've been stuffed with saliva-absorbing cotton. (The cure: drink water.)

COUCH-LOCK: The state of being too high to get off of the couch, typically found in smokers of heavy indica strains. A helpful mnemonic is that indica will leave you in-da-couch.

CREEPER: Weed with effects that sneak up on you, revealing themselves more slowly and subtly than immediate-head-rush strains, but packing a full punch in time. Among the strains identified as creepers: Strawberry Kush, Blueberry Diesel, and Chocolate Rain.

DARK SIDE OF THE RAINBOW: A classic stoner party trick, in which the 1939 film adaptation of *The Wizard of Oz* is screened on mute with subtitles, over a soundtrack of Pink Floyd's 1973 album *Dark Side of the Moon*, which, when started at the same time as the film, syncs up in a variety of seemingly meaningful ways with Dorothy's witch-bedeviled trip to the Emerald City. (For best results, start the album after the third roar of the MGM lion.)

EDIBLE DEATH LOOP: A hazardous trap in which people high on THC-enhanced food sate their munchies with more of the THC-enhanced food. Avoid at all costs. THC-spiked food is not food, it is medicine, even if it looks like the most delicious brownie in the world.

ENTOURAGE EFFECT: The habit of marijuana's sixty-plus cannabinoids to mix and mingle in unique ways to produce enhanced cumulative effects. (This is one **reason** why the few pharmaceutical drugs involving isolated THC, such as Marinol, can't compete with the cascading, complementary effects of actual marijuana.)

FATTY: A fat joint. "As soon as I finish performing **brain** surgery, I'm going to smoke a fatty."

GANJA: The Hindi word for marijuana, which should only be used by Hindis. (Take note, frat dudes in dreadlock **wigs.**)

GROW ROOM: A room devoted to the cultivation of marijuana, typically involving high-wattage lamps, ventilation fans, and, for careful growers, supplementary electrical generators. (High-wattage lamps require an unusual **amount** of electricity, and many a grow room has been busted after authorities followed the skyrocketing electricity bills.)

HASH: Also known as "hashish," hash is a marijuana product made of the plant's resin glands—those tiny crystally nubs (officially called trichomes) that form on flowering marijuana plants and pack a uniquely potent blast of cannabinoids. Depending on its preparation, hash can come in a variety of forms, from pressed solid blocks to gooey paste (sometimes called "bubble hash") to the dry-sift powder called kief. All of it will get you higher than normal marijuana.

HEAD SHOP: A retail store selling weed-friendly paraphernalia—pipes, bongs, vaporizers, pipe screens, rolling papers—all of which are typically presented as "tobacco accessories." (If you live in a prohibition state, don't mention weed in a head shop.)

HIGH TIMES: Founded in 1974 by Tom Forcade and published monthly ever since, *High Times* is the New York–based magazine devoted to the legalization of weed and the general celebration of weed culture. (Groovy fact: Past contributors include Charles Bukowski, William Burroughs, and Truman Capote.)

HOT BOX: The process of smoking marijuana in an enclosed space—typically a car with the windows rolled up, which clouds the air with secondhand smoke that is reinhaled and allegedly adds up to a stronger high. It also makes you smell like you're made entirely of weed, so smart hot-boxers take a long walk in fresh air before entering any rooms.

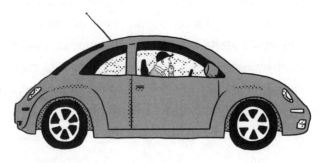

ICE BONG: A bong with ice placed in the chamber above the water, which further cools down the smoke before it enters the lungs. Some bongs have specific nubs built in to hold ice in the chamber above the lukewarm bong water, which is nice.

JACK HERER: American cannabis activist and author of *The Emperor Wears No Clothes*, a seminal book in the quest for sane marijuana, who founded and directed the organization Help End Marijuana Prohibition (HEMP) until his death in 2010.

MARIJUANA PARAPHERNALIA: Any product designed to facilitate the use of marijuana. Weed paraphernalia is typically split between user-based items (pipes, bongs, roach clips, rolling papers) and dealer-based items (scales, grow lights). Paraphernalia is sometimes used as probable cause to search for drugs. If you live in a prohibition state, hide your paraphernalia as conscientiously as you hide your weed.

MARY JANE: Slang term for weed that's essentially a honkified version of the Spanish word marijuana.

OPERATION PIPE DREAMS: Code name for the 2003 federal sting on retailers selling drug paraphernalia, with a specific eye on paraphernalia shipped over state lines. The most prominent victim: Tommy Chong, the legendary stoner comedian turned online pipe retailer, whose business was busted for mailing contraband, with Chong sentenced to nine months in federal prison. Galling twist: Federal prosecutors reportedly admitted to subjecting Chong to harsher-than-normal treatment in retaliation for his pot-loving, cop-mocking comedy.

THE RASTAFARI MOVEMENT: A religion started in Jamaica in the 1930s, the followers of which consider marijuana to be the Biblical Tree of Life, and use weed as a sacrament that brings them closer to God.

RICK SIMPSON: A medical marijuana patient in Canada who claims to have cured his cancer with cannabis oil, after which he set about helping others, supplying his marijuana oil medicine free to needy patients. These days, "Rick Simpson Oil" is a treasured product at legal medical marijuana dispensaries.

RIMONABANT: Earlier this century, a scientist was thinking about how weed gives users the munchies by triggering cannabinoid receptors connected to hunger. "What if there were a drug that didn't trigger but blocked hunger receptors?" this scientist person thought. "Would it maybe give people reverse-munchies and work as an anti-obesity drug?" The result was Rimombant, a drug that indeed blocked cannabinoid receptors but also made people susceptible to suicide, resulting in the drug's planned thirty-three-month study being abandoned after a year.

ROACH CLIP: A device used to hold joints when they've burned down to little nubs, allowing users to draw a last few puffs without burning their goddamn fingers.

SANJAY GUPTA: An American neurosurgeon and correspondent for CNN, who in 2013 identified himself as a medical-marijuana convert and apologized for his previous ignorance regarding weed's medical potential. As Gupta himself put it, "We have been terribly and systematically misled for nearly seventy years in the United States, and I apologize for my own role in that."

SEATTLE HEMPFEST: Held every summer on the Seattle waterfront, Hempfest is the world's largest annual event devoted to reforming America's pot laws, featuring bands, political speakers, and good-sport police officers. (After recreational weed was legalized in Washington, Seattle cops attended Hempfest to hand out mini-bags of Doritos inscribed with specifics of the new legal reality.)

SHAKE: Tiny flakes of weed that are the natural by-product of dealing with marijuana. Dealers typically sell shake at a lower price, and, if you're not the kind of person who cares about "dank bud" and "sticky weed," it works perfectly well at getting you high. Shake is particularly good for rolling joints (no grinding needed!) and making cannabutter.

SHOTGUN: A weed-smoking maneuver in which a person inhales from a pipe/bong/vaporizer/joint and exhales the smoke into someone else's mouth. (The exhaled smoke contains enough THC to justify the deed, and shotgunning someone you don't mind kissing is a bonus.)

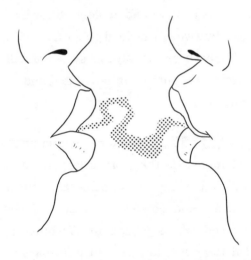

SMOKE OUT: To get someone high with your weed—either as repayment for a previous smoke out or just as a friendly gesture: "Thanks for loaning me your curling iron. Can I smoke you out?"

SYNTHETIC CANNABIS: Legal-for-now substances involving chemicals that mimic the effects of cannabis, which are sprayed onto non-cannabis plant material and sold under brand names like K2, Spice, and Spike. Synthetic cannabis occasionally drives people criminally insane and gives a whole bunch of other people monster headaches. Avoid.

TOKE: Slang for taking a draw on a pipe, bong, or joint: "Before we hit the fried cheese festival, let's have a toke."

WAKE AND BAKE: Rising from bed and promptly smoking weed. Good for rainy Saturdays filled with housecleaning, yard work, and Netflix. (Also good for alcohol hangovers.)

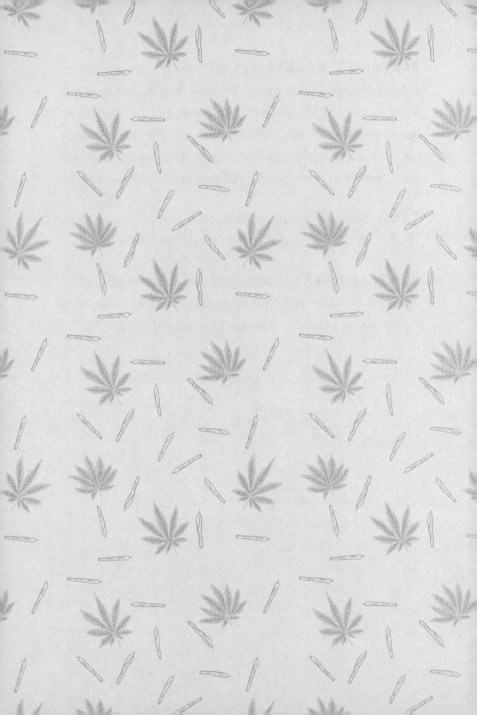

CLOSING NOTE: WHAT YOU NEED TO DO NOW

I live in a state that has fully legalized marijuana for recreational use, which is a wonderful thing. But any and all legal-weed wonderfulness remains tainted so long as our prisons hold those doing time—sometimes life sentences—for nonviolent marijuana convictions. So as I leave you, dear reader, I beg you to do three things:

1. Support any and all efforts to reclassify marijuana at the federal level. Simply moving marijuana from its severely restrictive Schedule 1 classification to a less restrictive Schedule 2 would enable lifesaving studies of marijuana's medical potential, while officially killing the notion that marijuana is a narcotic on par with heroin.

2. Do everything in your voting, marching, and letter-writing power to support an overhaul of marijuana sentencing laws, including the granting of clemency to those serving time for nonviolent marijuana convictions. As CNN's Mike Riggs wrote, "It should be cruel and unusual to mete out life-without-parole-sentences for a drug so mainstream that Colorado is using state-collected pot taxes to build new schools."

3. If/when you have an opportunity to vote in favor of legalized weed, do it. As pioneering pro-pot physician Dr. Lester Grinspoon wrote in the *Journal of the American Medical Association,* "The greatest danger in medical use of marijuana is its illegality, which imposes much anxiety and expense on suffering people, forces them to bargain with illicit drug dealers, and exposes them to the threat of criminal prosecution."

Then clean your bong and call your mother.

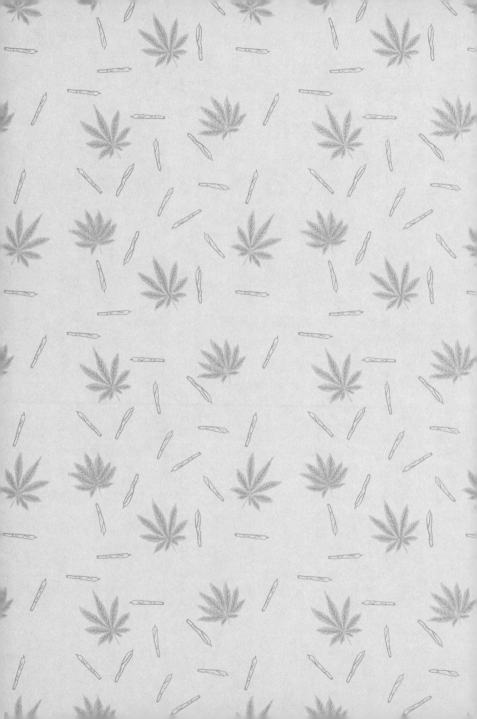

ACKNOWLEDGMENTS

Huge thanks to all the friends who helped me get this damn book done, especially recipe testers Mary Jarvis, Richard Kennedy, Jason Miller, Jaime Page, Adrian Ryan, and Bradley Steinbacher; draft readers Bethany Jean Clement, Gretchen Strauch, and Wally Schmader; and the many wonderful people who supplied me with marijuana over the years, including but not limited to Kent, Drewsky, Matthew, Chris, Todd, James, Waxy Brown, and Skillit. Final thanks to my husband, Jake Nelson, who is the world's funnest person to do everything with, including weed.

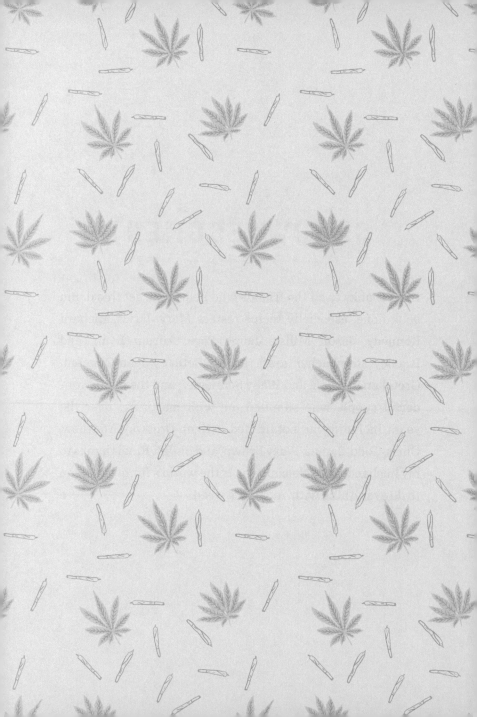

RESOURCES

GRASSCITY.COM: A virtual head shop selling pipes, bongs, vaporizers, grinders, rolling machines, cleaning supplies, and "420 lifestyle apparel." (This means T-shirts with pot leaves on them, not electric sweatpants that massage your legs while you watch *Murder, She Wrote.*)

LEAFLY.COM: A wealth of information about legal recreational marijuana, from detailed strain descriptions to a nationwide map of retail weed stores.

MARIJUANA ANONYMOUS: Want to stop (or cut back on) using marijuana and can't? You are not alone and the twelve step–based program Marijuana Anonymous is here to help, with online meetings, city-specific resources, and supportive chat rooms.
marijuana-anonymous.org

NORML: Want to join the fight to reform our country's disgraceful marijuana laws? NORML has been leading the charge for as long as there's been a charge, and their website features a wealth of ways for interested citizens to get involved.
norml.org

PROJECTCBD: A slew of valuable resources for doctors, patients, and policy makers interested in the medically potent but completely non-psychoactive cannabinoid CBD. **projectcbd.org**

PRONUNCIATION MANUAL: Go to youtu.be/Y31jRIhtvqo when you are high and want to laugh your face off. (Start with "haute couture," and listen to your heart from there.)

SOURCES

Brooklyn Public Library
CannaMagazine.com
High Times
Leafly
MedicalDaily.com
United Patients Group
Weedist

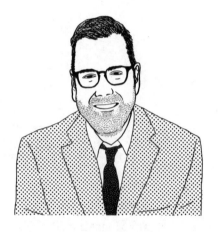

DAVID SCHMADER is a Texas-born writer and performer who has been living and working in Seattle since 1991. From 1999 to 2015, Schmader served as one of the defining voices of Seattle's Pulitzer-winning newsweekly the *Stranger*, writing the weekly pop culture and politics column Last Days. In his spare time, he's the world's foremost authority on the brilliant horribleness of the film *Showgirls*, hosting annotated screenings across the country and supplying the commentary track for the best-selling *Showgirls* DVD.

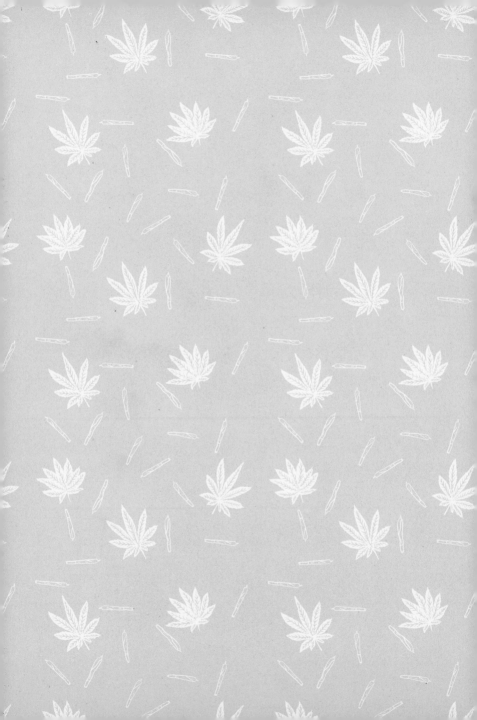